Dr. Lytle's extensive experience in designing, developing, and evaluating multilevel behavioral interventions is the foundation for this important and timely book for researchers and practitioners. She has been the lead on many successful interventions involving youth and adults concerning multiple health problems and associated behaviors, and this has resulted in a framework based on science and achievement. Her clarity reflects this wealth of knowledge, and she gifts us with clear and cogent steps to making our communities healthier places.

—**Cheryl L. Perry, PhD,** Professor Emerita, Department of Health Promotion and Behavioral Sciences, University of Texas Health Science Center at Houston; School of Public Health, Austin Campus, Austin, TX, United States

Leslie Lytle has written a practical guide for how to plan theoretically sound, creative, and effective policies and interventions to promote healthy behaviors. Concrete examples take the reader through the various steps of the process. The book is systematic and engaging—highly recommended!

—**Knut-Inge Klepp, PhD,** Executive Director, Norwegian Institute of Public Health, Oslo, Norway

This is an excellent resource for students, researchers, and practitioners. The stepwise process for creating, implementing, and evaluating multilevel interventions is clearly described and easy to follow. Dr. Lytle's decades-long experience with designing and evaluating multilevel interventions is made evident through her practical guidance and applied intervention examples.

—**Jess Haines, PhD, MHSc, RD,** Department of Family Relations and Applied Nutrition, University of Guelph, Guelph, Ontario, Canada

Designing Interventions to Promote Community Health

Designing Interventions to Promote Community Health

| A Multilevel, Stepwise Approach |

Leslie Ann Lytle

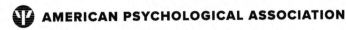
AMERICAN PSYCHOLOGICAL ASSOCIATION

Published by
American Psychological Association
750 First Street, NE
Washington, DC 20002
https://www.apa.org

Order Department
https://www.apa.org/pubs/books
order@apa.org

In the U.K., Europe, Africa, and the Middle East, copies may be ordered from Eurospan
https://www.eurospanbookstore.com/apa
info@eurospangroup.com

Typeset in Meridien and Ortodoxa by Circle Graphics, Inc., Reisterstown, MD

Printer: Gasch Printing, Odenton, MD
Cover Designer: Nicci Falcone, Potomac, MD

Library of Congress Cataloging-in-Publication Data

Names: Lytle, Leslie A., author.
Title: Designing interventions to promote community health : a multilevel, stepwise approach / by Leslie A. Lytle.
Description: Washington, DC : American Psychological Association, [2022] | Includes bibliographical references and index.
Identifiers: LCCN 2022002431 (print) | LCCN 2022002432 (ebook) | ISBN 9781433836503 (paperback) | ISBN 9781433838026 (ebook)
Subjects: LCSH: Health promotion. | Community health services. | BISAC: MEDICAL / Public Health | SOCIAL SCIENCE / Disease & Health Issues
Classification: LCC RA427.8 .L98 2022 (print) | LCC RA427.8 (ebook) | DDC 362.1--dc23/eng/20220404
LC record available at https://lccn.loc.gov/2022002431
LC ebook record available at https://lccn.loc.gov/2022002432

https://doi.org/10.1037/0000292-000

Printed in the United States of America

10 9 8 7 6 5 4 3 2 1

*This book is dedicated to my family and friends
who have added abundant joy to my journey.*

CONTENTS

ACKNOWLEDGMENTS

I greatly appreciate the insights, feedback, and support that I received from colleagues who reviewed drafts of this book. In particular, I thank Cheryl Perry, Susan Ennett, Vangie Foshee, Alexandra Lightfoot, and Allison Myers for their feedback on the Introduction and the Plan and Create Phases. Stacey Moe and Kristen Polzien gave useful feedback on the Implement Phase from their perspectives as project coordinators. David Murray and June Stevens offered important advice on the Evaluate Phase, and Jennifer Leeman and Ross Brownson reviewed the chapter on adapting interventions. Gretchen Musicant, Kristen Klingler, and Lara Pratt from the Minneapolis Health Department provided insights on how practitioners approach the task of designing community-based interventions. Everyone that I approached for help was so gracious and generous with their time; I am truly honored to have such wonderful colleagues and friends. Thanks also to the three anonymous reviewers. Your insights strengthened the book. Finally, thank you to Susan Reynolds and David Becker from the American Psychological Association. Susan reached out to me to write this book, and David served as development editor. It was a delight to work with both of you.

A special note of gratitude to my two mentors, Cheryl Perry and David Murray. Since my earliest days as a postdoc in the Division of Epidemiology at the University of Minnesota, you both have guided, supported, and encouraged me. You both have made me laugh—a lot! Most important, you have shown me that exceptional scientists and successful academicians can also be kind and caring people with full and rich lives. I am eternally grateful to you both.

Designing Interventions to Promote Community Health

Introduction

Changing behavior is incredibly difficult. Consider the times that you vowed to eat a healthier diet, get more exercise or more sleep, floss your teeth daily, drink less alcohol, or quit smoking. Even you, someone reading a book about designing interventions to change behavior, likely finds behavior change difficult.

In the United States, three health behaviors (smoking cigarettes, not getting enough physical activity, and eating the wrong kinds of foods or too much food) are responsible for nearly 75% of the variability in life expectancy through their impact on the prevalence of obesity, diabetes, and hypertension (Dwyer-Lindgren et al., 2017). Beyond these "big three," many other health behaviors contribute to the burden of disease in the United States and globally, including drinking and driving, hygiene related to the spread of infectious disease, engaging in unprotected sex, aggressive and violent behavior, poor adherence to medication regimens, and ignoring advice regarding preventive care.

There is an urgent need for effective and efficient health behavior change interventions to reduce the burden of disease. But how do we design interventions to maximize their potential to be effective in facilitating behavior change? How do we plan for and create interventions with sustainability and dissemination in mind? What needs to be considered as we implement interventions to make sure that they are delivered as intended and can be replicated by others? How do we evaluate these interventions so we can demonstrate their effectiveness and learn as much as possible about how they work, for whom

https://doi.org/10.1037/0000292-001
Designing Interventions to Promote Community Health: A Multilevel, Stepwise Approach,
by L. A. Lytle

they work, and how to improve upon them? How are interventions adapted to meet the needs of specific populations?

WHAT IS THE PURPOSE OF THIS BOOK?

The purpose of this book is to provide a stepwise process for designing multilevel behavior change interventions to promote community health. My use of the word "design" encompasses a consideration of all of the phases of developing a behavior change intervention, including how a team plans, creates, implements, and evaluates the intervention. The focus of the book is on designing new multilevel interventions (MLIs), but the process suggested may be helpful to those adapting existing evidence-based intervention (EBIs) by providing a systematic approach for making decisions about what adaptations are required to meet the needs of a community.

Multilevel interventions attempt to change not only individual behavior but also the places and systems that provide the context within which individual behavioral choices are made. Because behavior change is so difficult, targeting change at multiple levels increases the chance that the intervention will be effective. Because a multilevel approach targets system change as well as individual change, the chance that the intervention will be sustainable is increased. This book groups the contexts that influence health behavior into three environmental levels: individual, social, and physical environments. These three environmental levels provide the framework for designing MLIs.

The emphasis of the book is on designing health behavior programs using a community-engaged approach. A community-engaged approach includes community stakeholders in all stages of the intervention design. The importance of involving community speaks to the need to create interventions that meet the needs of the community, embrace community assets, reflect and respect community culture, and build community capacity. Engaging community throughout the process increases the chances that the intervention will be acceptable, feasible, and sustainable.

The intervention design approach is intended for health problems that are widespread in the community that can either be prevented by engaging in healthy behaviors (universal prevention) or remediated through behavior changes (selective prevention). The process and examples used throughout the book reflect my public health perspective and experience as a behavioral scientist creating and evaluating MLIs in community settings. However, increasingly, medical systems are developing and offering behavior change programs for their clinic populations and may find the process detailed in this book useful.

WHO IS THE AUDIENCE FOR THIS BOOK?

The audience for this book includes both researchers and practitioners who are designing or adapting behavior change programs to improve population health. Students preparing to enter a health profession as researchers or practitioners will find the book useful as a blueprint for guiding their work. In addition, researchers and health professionals already working in the areas of public health, community health, occupational health, nursing, and medicine who are developing new community-based interventions or adapting EBIs to meet the needs of their own community will find the information and suggestions herein useful. This book's contents will be particularly valuable to the behavioral scientists or program planners who are responsible for creating the content and activities that will make up the intervention.

Creating and evaluating the effectiveness of behavioral interventions through a rigorously designed intervention trial is typically the work of researchers. Intervention trials are time-constrained; their beginning and ending is predetermined by a funding mechanism. Therefore, clarity of purpose and a process for planning and creating the intervention are crucial from the beginning of the trial. The intervention must be able to be implemented with rigor and according to a protocol that allows details of the intervention to be replicated. The research team must plan for an evaluation that helps them determine if their intervention was effective in creating behavioral change, as well as understand how and for whom the intervention worked. This book details the process for designing interventions to be evaluated in research settings using rigorous intervention trials.

Practitioners, on the other hand, may use a variety of approaches in program planning. They may develop their own interventions based on community wisdom, or they may adapt EBIs with proven effectiveness in other communities. Many EBIs will need to be modified to be culturally appropriate for a specific community, adapted to meet implementation challenges unique to a community, and refined to make sure that evaluation tools and metrics meet the needs of the community. This volume offers insights into how the phases and steps outlined may be used by those adapting existing interventions. Although practitioners may not be conducting rigorous intervention trials, they will want to be able to evaluate their programs to ascertain whether outcomes can be attributed to the intervention efforts and to understand how, and for whom, the intervention worked. This book provides information on conducting formative, process, and outcome evaluations that will be valuable to both researchers and practitioners.

WHAT APPROACH IS USED?

The theory-informed approach in these pages was adapted from an intervention planning process created by Perry (1999). The book guides the user through the process of designing an MLI using a stepwise approach organized by phases. This organization is not meant to be a strict recipe (there is invariably a cyclical nature to the process) but a guidepost to help keep intervention teams focused on important tasks. Twelve steps are organized within four phases:

The Plan Phase

1. Identify a behavior-based community health problem.
2. Choose the relevant behavioral determinants.

3. Create a conceptual model.
4. Review the conceptual model with the evaluation team and community stakeholders.

The Create Phrase

5. Write the intervention objectives and identify potential intervention components.
6. Design intervention strategies.
7. Create a logic model.
8. Share the logic model with the evaluation team and community stakeholders.

The Implement Phrase

9. Develop process evaluation measures.
10. Finalize intervention protocol, training, and materials.

The Evaluate Phase

11. Evaluate the effectiveness of the intervention.
12. Prepare for the next iteration or dissemination of the intervention.

The book will not provide every detail needed to plan, create, implement, and evaluate interventions; additional resources and expertise will be needed. Important considerations regarding how to find funding for community-based interventions, the process of community engagement, and the ethical issues related to working in and with community are beyond the scope of this book. In addition, a team designing a community-based behavior change intervention will need expertise in study design and biostatistics.

There is a growing recognition that no one theory holds the key to understanding behavior change. A chapter is included that reviews health behavior theories that help identify determinants or predictors of behavior (a key step in the Plan Phase) as well as health behavior theories that focus on how change happens (the focus of the Create Phase). Information on theory is presented in a way that stresses its practical use to those designing interventions or programs.

Currently, there is great interest in *implementation science*, a broad term that includes the development and application of common principles, models, and designs to understand and promote the uptake of EBIs (Brownson et al., 2015). Implementation science begins with the assumption that there are interventions or intervention approaches that have demonstrated effectiveness and efficacy and are ready to be adopted by other communities and populations. Implementation science deals with how to facilitate the dissemination and implementation process so that effective interventions can extend their reach. The goal of this book is to help teams across the globe develop interventions that are effective, efficacious, and community-centric, thereby increasing the number of EBIs for dissemination. The approach that I propose engages communities in all phases of the intervention design with an intention of designing interventions that will be relevant to communities, feasible to implement in communities, and create value within communities. Those attributes promote the sustainability of the intervention as well as its dissemination to other communities.

OVERVIEW OF THE BOOK'S CONTENTS

The book begins with a discussion of MLIs in Chapter 1, including what they are, why they are useful, and the utility and limitations of ecological models in developing multilevel interventions. Next, a framework for MLIs that focus on changes at the individual, social, and physical environments is presented, followed by an example of an MLI. Chapter 1 concludes with an overview of the four phases of the design process, including a summary of each of the 12 steps. Chapter 2 reviews theories of behavior change and includes theories addressing change at the individual level and theories addressing system-level or organizational change. The focus is on a practical application of theory, with a distinction made between theories that help identify the factors that are related to behaviors and theories that suggest the mechanisms of how change happens, both in individuals and in organizations. Chapters 3 through 6 describe how to implement the four phases and corresponding steps of the multilevel design process, with each chapter representing one phase: Chapter 3 describes the Plan Phase, Chapter 4 the Create Phase, Chapter 5 the Implement Phase, and Chapter 6 the Evaluate Phase. To illustrate the steps in each phase, I develop a hypothetical intervention with the goal of reducing middle-school students' consumption of sugar-sweetened beverages. Finally, Chapter 7 provides guidelines for adapting existing interventions to different communities by using a modified version of the four-phase multilevel design framework.

SUMMARY

Changing behavior is a very difficult task, and no framework, set of steps, or process can guarantee success. We still need to learn a great deal about how to positively influence health behavior change in communities, sustain change, and adapt interventions to meet the ever-changing needs of the population and the fluid environments that have an impact on our behaviors. Although following the steps in this book cannot guarantee success, using the framework and process described will help prevent avoidable mistakes, enhance what we can learn from our attempts, and keep us grounded in our purpose of improving the health of communities.

As a final note, this book was written during the global pandemic caused by COVID-19. The epidemic has highlighted the great importance of health behavior in preventing and mitigating disease risk. People around the globe have received instructions on how to wash their hands, the importance of wearing masks, and the need to practice social distancing. People have been encouraged to be vaccinated in order to reduce their risk of COVID-19 and reduce community transmission. Individual behavior, supported by a change in community norms, is a primary mechanism for reducing the spread of this deadly virus. This pandemic is not just about health behavior related to infectious disease, however. As we search for the underlying factors that make some more vulnerable to COVID-19, preexisting health conditions, including obesity, diabetes, and heart disease, are showing up as potentially important risk factors. The vast majority of these preexisting conditions have their genesis in health behavior and are influenced by organizational, systemic, and market-driven forces. The COVID-19 pandemic is also highlighting the influence of health disparities on morbidity and mortality as communities of color and vulnerable and low-income communities suffer disproportionately, both health-wise and economically. It is my hope that we emerge from this pandemic with a deeper commitment to the health and well-being of all people and to a recalibration of the systems that influence our behavioral choices.

1

A Multilevel Framework for Intervention Design

Overview of the Phases and Steps

In this chapter, I begin by discussing the utility of multilevel interventions (MLIs) to promote community health, and I describe the importance of MLIs in tackling complex public health problems, such as smoking, diet, and physical activity. Although social ecological models are frequently used in public health, they have some important limitations when used to design MLIs. I introduce the framework that I use throughout the book to guide the design of an MLI that organizes determinants that impact behavior by environments described in ecological models, specifically, individual, social, and physical environments. This chapter includes an explanation of the types of behavioral determinants found at each environmental level and an overview of how they are measured. The framework also suggests a causal path between the determinants and the target behavior to guide evaluation planning and hypothesis testing. I provide an example of an MLI that was rigorously evaluated and widely disseminated. Next, I introduce the phases and steps that will be used to guide the process of designing a behavior change intervention: the Plan, Create, Implement, and Evaluate Phases. Included in this chapter are definitions for terms that I use frequently throughout this volume.

https://doi.org/10.1037/0000292-002
Designing Interventions to Promote Community Health: A Multilevel, Stepwise Approach,
by L. A. Lytle

WHAT ARE MULTILEVEL INTERVENTIONS, AND WHY ARE THEY USEFUL?

The focus of traditional health behavior interventions is to change individuals. Traditional health interventions attempt to achieve change by providing individuals with knowledge about the consequences of their behavior, convincing them that the benefits they would realize by changing their behavior would outweigh the costs of change, helping them identify the cues and reinforcements of their behaviors, teaching them new skills related to enacting the new behavior (e.g., how to prepare a healthy snack or establish a healthy sleep environment), and teaching them skills related to behavior management (e.g., self-monitoring, goal setting, self-reinforcement). Interventions focusing on individual behavior change can be delivered to individuals or groups, and the intervention approaches typically used include health education, health communication and campaigns, and individual and group counseling sessions. App-based interventions that attempt to provide information, motivate, cue behaviors, provide opportunities to monitor one's behavior, and reinforce behavioral responses are examples of individual-level interventions. Implied in this approach (but often not explicitly stated) is that once change occurs, it will persist, healthy patterns and habits will be established, and health will ensue. However, these traditional behavior change approaches are seldom successful in the long term, especially with complex behaviors that require daily decision making and when one's social and physical environment makes it challenging to make the healthy behavioral choice.

More recently, attention has turned from individual-level, downstream approaches toward upstream approaches that focus on impacting the context in which behavioral choices are made. Behavioral decisions do not occur in a vacuum but rather reflect the traditions, culture, norms, and behaviors of those around us. Likewise, individual choice may be limited—and certainly influenced—by the physical environment that individuals are exposed to in their daily life. Social, political, and economic systems that are beyond the immediate control of individuals affect behavioral choices. Therefore, instead of relying on health campaigns encouraging people to walk more, upstream intervention approaches focus on designing communities with sidewalks, crosswalks, and more green space. Likewise, instead of using nutrition education to convince people that they should eat healthier foods, upstream efforts have shifted to bringing more full-service grocery stores into food deserts (i.e., urban areas where it can be difficult to find affordable, good-quality food) and expanding the healthy offerings in corner stores.

Upstream approaches attempt to instigate change in the larger social, economic, political, and physical environmental levels as a way to improve population health (McKinlay & Marceau, 1999). These intervention approaches include legislative, regulatory, economic, policy, and practice changes that have an impact on large segments of the population. Upstream approaches often focus on influencing the social and physical environments. For example, a schoolwide policy that bans vaping at school is an upstream approach targeting the social environment, whereas city zoning that requires the addition of lighted sidewalks is an upstream approach targeting the physical environment.

Upstream approaches alone may not be sufficient to influence population behavior, however. For complex behaviors, such as eating and physical activity, it appears that effecting change at multiple levels is required for sustained change and improved population health. As an example, the STORE (STaple foods ORdinance Evaluation) Study used the enactment of a city ordinance requiring licensed grocery stores to carry a set of healthy staple foods as a natural experiment to evaluate the effectiveness of the policy to have an impact on both the foods available in stores and consumer behavior. Using another city as a comparison group, audits and consumer intercept surveys (i.e., surveys conducted with consumers as they exit a store) were conducted before and after the implementation of the policy. More healthy foods were offered in the stores in both cities over time, but no significant differences in change were evident between the two cities; the impact appeared to be a secular change rather than a result of the city ordinance. Importantly, there was little or no evidence of change in consumer behavior within or between cities (Laska et al., 2019). While a natural experiment such as this has some limitations as a study design, results suggest that an opportunity in the physical environment is a necessary—but not sufficient—condition for change. Likewise, research has consistently shown that people's perceptions of their local food environment—specifically, foods available in their neighborhood stores and the prices of healthy foods available—do not match what is actually available in their environment.

THE SUCCESS OF MULTILEVEL INTERVENTIONS ON THE "BIG THREE" HEALTH BEHAVIORS: SMOKING, DIET, AND PHYSICAL ACTIVITY

Of the three behaviors most responsible for the burden of disease in the United States, smoking is the only one that has been decreasing in prevalence over the past decades (Office of Disease Prevention and Health Promotion, n.d.). This public health success is likely due to a synergy of both downstream and upstream approaches, including tobacco price increases, antitobacco mass-media campaigns, comprehensive smoke-free laws, and increased access to smoking cessation programs. Similar success with population-level changes in healthy eating and physical activity has not yet been realized, despite national guidelines explicitly stating the risks and advocating for change (U.S. Department of Health and Human Services, 2018; U.S. Department of Agriculture, 2020). The lack of progress in changing these behaviors is likely due to the challenges faced in enacting upstream policy approaches that affect food availability and pricing (Nestle, 2013) and the slow process of urban planning and revitalization (Mayne et al., 2015). With food and activity patterns being part of every culture and social group, changing social norms regarding eating and activity behaviors is especially challenging.

In addition, people's perceptions of what is available in the environment appear to predict their behavior better than what is actually present in the environment (Giskes et al., 2007).

Increasingly, there is an awareness that to change health behaviors, interventions must intentionally plan to spark change at more than one level of influence. These MLIs (also called *complex interventions*; Hawe, 2015) recognize that the context within which one makes behavioral choices is important not only to understand but also, when possible, to intervene upon.

The use of MLI approaches over single-level approaches has many advantages. Making individuals responsible for change in an unsupportive environment puts the burden of change squarely on the shoulders of the individual. MLIs have the potential to reduce victim blaming and provide support to individuals as they attempt to change behavior. In addition, by changing aspects of the social or physical environment, positive environments can be created for the entire community, not just those who seek care. Doing so helps normalize, incentivize, and reinforce healthier behavioral options for all exposed. MLIs may be uniquely suited to reducing health disparities because of the emphasis on system-level change working to influence organizations, policies, practices, places, and social systems (Gorin et al., 2012). Change occurring at a higher level of influence has a better chance of sustainability and long-term impact than does change that rests solely at the individual level. Finally, MLIs are, by nature, transdisciplinary, meaning that stakeholders with a variety of expertise need to be involved in planning, creating, implementing, and evaluating the intervention. This diversity of knowledge and experience allows for interventions that are more complex and nuanced and better suited to a given community, reflecting the reality within which behavior happens and the possibility for change to occur.

In 2012, the *Journal of the National Cancer Institute Monographs* released a set of articles describing and detailing elements of MLIs. In the Introduction, an *intervention* is defined as a "specified strategy or set of strategies, designed to change the knowledge, perceptions, skills and/or behaviors of individuals, groups, or organizations, with the goal of improving health outcomes" (Taplin et al., 2012, p. 3). The authors of another article in the monograph defined MLIs as interventions designed to influence more than one contextual level— including individuals as well as groups, organizations, and the community (Clauser et al., 2012). Although the emphasis of their commentary is on the utility of MLIs applied to health care delivery, the application of MLIs is relevant to all public health interventions, including those designed to promote health and prevent disease.

THE UTILITY AND LIMITATIONS OF ECOLOGICAL MODELS IN CREATING MULTILEVEL INTERVENTIONS

Ecological models are graphic representations of the relationship between an individual and their environment and are helpful in representing the myriad contexts that may influence an individual's behavior. The earliest ecological model was posed by Urie Bronfenbrenner (1992) to explain how the environments that a child is exposed to (e.g., family, school, cultural values, customs) interact with the unique characteristics of the child to impact growth and development. Ecological models have been adapted and expanded over time to provide insights into complex public health problems. As an example, Story et al. (2008) suggested an ecological model to portray the various influences on childhood obesity. Using a system of concentric circles, individual factors including cognitions and skills are at the innermost circle, representing the most proximal influence on obesity risk. That inner circle is surrounded, in turn, by circles representing the social (networks), physical (settings), and macro (sectors) environments. The model suggests specific attributes of each layer that influence obesity risk. For example, family and friends provide influence at the social environment level through role modeling and social support related to eating behavior and activity choices, while attributes of the physical environment (including home, school, and neighborhood features) influence access, availability, opportunities and barriers to eating and activity choices. The macro environment includes government and political structures, as well as the food industry, all of which influence behavioral choices and obesity risk through policy and legislative actions. In addition, social ecological models are used globally to understand a wide range of public health problems, including UNICEF's (2017) use of an ecological model to improve the health of children by reducing cholera, increasing breastfeeding, and reducing malnutrition or the World Health Organization's (n.d.) use of an ecological framework as part of the Global Campaign for Violence Prevention.

While ecological models are important heuristics for understanding the many influences on population health, they have some important limitations. It is not possible to design an intervention that will have a positive impact across all settings that make up the physical environment or all the social networks that influence one's behavior. Rarely is there time or funding to effect change at the macrolevel. Interventionists need to make choices about what factors should be the focus of their interventions; an ecological model suggests that all factors are potentially important. For example, an ecological model suggests that worksites may be an important venue related to obesity risk for adults, but it does not suggest which aspects of the worksite will be important to address in an intervention. Should intervention efforts focus on the lack of access to exercise options onsite during or after work, or should they focus on the social norms of the worksite encouraging donut and cookie breaks? Another limitation of ecological models is that they do not suggest causal relationships. In evaluating the impact of MLIs, there is a need to specify the behavioral outcome that will be used to evaluate the effectiveness of the intervention and to identify a discrete number of exposures or determinants that will be targeted to create change in the outcome. Although determinants at different levels of influence are expected to interact, patterns of influence and assumption of causality need be considered a priori to design an evaluation plan to assess the effectiveness of an intervention.

A FRAMEWORK FOR MULTILEVEL INTERVENTIONS

The framework that I will use for developing MLIs organizes behavioral determinants by the environments described in an ecological model: individual,
social, and physical environments (Figure 1.1). These three environments
become the levels making up an MLI. The framework shows a causal model
in which the social, physical, and individual environments have reciprocal
effects on each other environmental level and direct and indirect influences
on a specific health behavior. A biological health outcome is included in the
framework because, as health professionals, we care about influencing health
behavior in order to reduce population health disease risk, but the focus of
the intervention is on changing behaviors and behavioral determinants. The
framework also suggests potential modifying factors to consider. Modifying
factors are not on the causal pathway suggested in the framework. They may
include covariates and confounding variables to be included in the analysis to
reduce bias. They may also include potential moderators that affect relationships in the model. Modifying factors may include factors at the individual
level, such as genetics and biology, as well as sociodemographic characteristics,
including age, gender, race/ethnicity, income, and educational level. Modifying
factors may also occur at the neighborhood level, including the racial and ethnic
diversity of the community, whether the neighborhood is in an urban or rural
area, its population size and density, and the mean household income of the
community. Although modifying factors are not directly addressed through
a behavior change intervention, the sociodemographic characteristics of the
individuals targeted in the intervention may affect both their participation in
and response to the intervention. In addition, neighborhood characteristics
influence the behavioral options and opportunities in a community. The extent
to which these modifying factors can be measured and included in analytic
models will enhance what can be learned about the effectiveness and potential of a community-based intervention.

Determinants From the Individual Environment

The determinants or factors that are most proximally related to a health behavior
and most directly influence behavioral choices are those from the individual
environment. In this book, I use the term *individual environment* to characterize
the determinants that are inherent to the individual; I think of the individual
environment as the "environment between the ears." Those determinants
include knowledge, attitudes, values, behavioral skills, self-efficacy, habits and
preferences, and perceptions. Knowledge, attitudes, and values include what
one knows and understands about how to be healthy and how much one values
health in relationship to other things that are important. Behavioral skills are
required to enact many health behaviors, whereas self-efficacy represents one's
confidence in their ability to use those behavioral skills. As an example, to quit
smoking, several behavioral skills need to be learned, such as how to manage
stress and reduce cues for smoking. In addition to having those skills, one must

FIGURE 1.1. Framework for Designing Multilevel Interventions

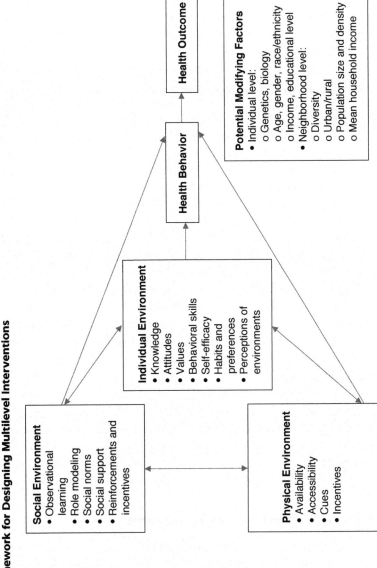

also feel confident that they can use those skills when the urge to smoke occurs. Having skills to make changes and feeling self-efficacious about one's ability to make those changes increase the chances that an individual will respond by resisting the urge to smoke when presented with a cue to do so. The individual environment is formed by one's life experience and reflects past learning and behavioral preferences that have become habituated over time. Habits are those behaviors that are so well established that no ongoing decision making occurs. Preferences may be both innate and learned, influenced by genetics as well as what is learned through experience with the larger environment. The individual environment also includes one's perceptions of the physical and social environment.

Determinants From the Social Environment

Influence from the social environment may come from people who are close to us, such as our family, friends, coworkers, and neighbors, or from more distal sources, such as social media, the larger culture, including movies and marketing, and rules and policies that shape social interaction in the larger environment. The social environment may influence behaviors through both subtle and direct means. Observational or vicarious learning happens when we watch others behave and observe how their behaviors are reinforced. For example, if a friend begins to walk regularly to reduce her stress and she appears more relaxed, I may learn vicariously that walking has some positive benefits. Role models in the social environment are particularly powerful in influencing behavior when we perceive those role models to be like us. These subtle influences also help to establish social norms for behavior. An obvious example of social norms is the importance that parents play as role models for their children. Parental behaviors teach the child much more about how to behave than does parental advice. "Do what I say and not what I do" is not a successful parental strategy for teaching children how to behave.

The social environment can also include direct influences on behavior through the provision of social support, tangible reinforcements, and incentives to behave in a certain way. Community health leaders and peer support networks can directly affect the social environment through the provision of social support for those needing help. Worksite wellness programs that provide discounts to fitness centers are using tangible reinforcements to incentivize workers' activity.

Determinants From the Physical Environment

The physical environment includes determinants in physical spaces (including homes, schools, worksites, community centers, clinics, neighborhoods, and retail spaces) that enable or promote behaviors. I think of the physical environment as places without people. This physical environment includes the availability and accessibility of behavioral options as well as behavioral cues and incentives in the physical space. *Availability* refers to the presence or absence of a behavioral option, while *accessibility* adds the dimension of being able to access that option.

As examples, fresh fruit may be available in a neighborhood store, but its price limits my ability to buy—or access—that fruit. I may want to be vaccinated for shingles, but lack of availability of the vaccine in my neighborhood prohibits me from acting on that choice. There may be a park in my neighborhood, but it is not accessible to me because of my concerns about safety. Examples of behavioral cues include labeling products as healthy in the grocery store or signs that encourage people to use the stairs, while incentives in the physical environment might be signs offering a two-for-one promotional sale.

The categorization of these three environments (individual, social, and physical) as unique, independent influences on behavior is a contrived representation designed for simplicity. These environments interact constantly in fluid and organic ways. As examples, I may be inclined to buy apples because of the signage in the store, but my child who is shopping with me may convince me that cookies are the better choice. The lack of availability of shingles vaccinations in my area may be circumvented by a neighbor who tells me where vaccinations are available nearby and stresses the importance of getting vaccinated. My perception that my neighborhood is not safe to walk may not be supported

EXAMPLES OF HOW ATTRIBUTES FROM EACH ENVIRONMENT ARE MEASURED

More details on how determinants from the individual, social, and physical environments are measured are included in Chapter 6, which covers the Evaluate Phase. A brief review of the most typical methods for evaluating each environment follows.

- **Individual environment** is typically assessed by asking the individual to report on what they know, believe, think, feel, or experience and occurs using surveys, questionnaires, or interviews. Behavioral skills can be assessed using self-monitoring or through direct observation.

- **Social environment** can be assessed by observing or documenting the behaviors of one's social networks or the behaviors of other people to whom an individual is exposed. For example, documenting the proportion of teachers who drink sugar-sweetened beverages during the school day is a way to assess the role-modeling around beverage choice to which students are exposed. Social network analysis and dyadic analysis are other measurement methods to assess the social environment.

- **Physical environment** can be assessed through audits or inventories that use observation to document availability, accessibility, cues, and incentives. A geographic information system (GIS) is a commonly used tool for documenting the built environment, defined as the manmade structures, features, and facilities viewed collectively as environments in which people live and work and is used for integrating and analyzing spatial and geographic data.

by any objective police or community-level data and may change if I observe others enjoying being outside.

The interaction between levels is reflected in the framework in two ways. First, the interaction between the three environments is represented using bidirectional lines linking each level, suggesting that change in any one environment may impact the others. In addition, while the framework suggests that each environment has a direct effect on behavior, it also shows that the social and physical environments have indirect effects that are mediated by the individual environment. This indirect effect points to the importance one's perceptions of their social and physical environments has for their behavioral choices. Much

HOW DOES THE MACROLEVEL ENVIRONMENT FIT IN WITH DESIGNING INTERVENTIONS?

It is undeniable that macrolevel forces have the greatest influence on the health of populations (Marmot, 2015). The macro environment includes the influence of social and structural factors that influence population health, including structural racism and inherent bias in policies and practices and includes the systems in place that support the status quo. The ability to earn a living wage, get an education, have access to affordable housing and health care, to be able to buy healthy foods at a reasonable price, and to be treated fairly and respectfully are conditions that either give tremendous advantage or pose incredible challenges to health. These macrolevel factors influence morbidity and mortality risk directly as well as through the opportunities or challenges that they bring to the enactment of health-related behaviors.

Working to positively influence the macrolevel environment is incredibly important. However, attempting to change the macrolevel environment is beyond the scope of most behavioral interventions and practice-based programs. Changes at the macrolevel often require enactment of state or federal policy or legislation as well as larger cultural or societal shifts that take decades or even generations to achieve. Intervention research and program initiatives occurring in the community are typically not able to directly intervene at the macrolevel. With this acknowledgment, factors at the macrolevel are immensely important in determining the individual, social, and physical environments that each of us must navigate. Macrolevel forces must be considered as we seek to design health behavior change interventions to improve the health of communities. As health professionals, it is essential to be respectful of the communities that we work with, learn about and appreciate their history, and acknowledge community assets. In addition, we can look for ways to build on the strengths of the communities that we work with by inviting them to the table as partners, providing training, employing members of the community to work on projects, and developing programs and interventions that will help improve all aspects of health, including physical, social, and mental health. Working to intervene on the ways in which macrolevel forces differentially distribute harmful exposures and finding ways to help all people reach their potential is the work of a lifetime.

more complicated statistical modeling can be done to examine the influence of each environment and determinant on the behavioral outcome, but for the purpose of designing behavioral interventions, the simplicity of this framework provides a useful blueprint and a way to organize and consider the most relevant factors related to a health outcome. The framework is also useful as a way to emphasize the importance of intervening across multiple environments to create synergy between them.

AN EXAMPLE OF A MULTILEVEL INTERVENTION: CATCH

The Child and Adolescent Trial for Cardiovascular Health (CATCH; Luepker et al., 1996; Perry et al., 1990) is an example of an MLI. CATCH was a school-based intervention trial funded by the National Institutes of Health in the early 1990s with a goal of reducing the risk of future cardiovascular disease in elementary school–age children. CATCH was a universal prevention, group- or cluster-randomized community trial conducted in 96 schools in four states. The CATCH intervention occurred in a cohort of students during their third-through fifth-grade years. CATCH was designed to assess change in serum cholesterol in children exposed to the intervention compared with children in the control group; that change was expected to occur through improvements in students' dietary intake (specifically, change in total fat, saturated fat, and sodium) and increased levels of physical activity.

The CATCH intervention was designed to have an effect on determinants influencing the eating and activity behaviors of youth at the individual, social, and physical environments using classroom curricula, changes in school food service, and changes in physical education class as intervention components. CATCH included classroom curricula in all three grades: Hearty Heart and Friends (third grade), Go for Health 4 (fourth grade), and Go for Health 5 (fifth grade). Each curriculum included activities designed to change student-level knowledge, attitudes, and skills regarding making healthy diet and activity choices. Curricular content also included knowledge, attitudes, and skills to prevent the initiation of smoking. Although the focus of the curricula was on the individual environment, aspects of the social environment were also positively affected by the CATCH curricular component through the classroom activities that promoted role-modeling of healthy behaviors.

The Eat Smart school cafeteria component was designed with school food service managers and staff to influence the physical and social environments of school cafeterias. At the physical environment level, Eat Smart worked with school food service staff to change menu options and modify recipes to reduce the amount of total fat, saturated fat, and sodium in foods served in school lunch. In addition, the Eat Smart component included helping food service staff market the new lower fat and lower sodium foods on the menu through promotions and signage. To influence the social environment, Eat Smart encouraged school staff to reinforce healthy choices through their interactions with students as they went through the cafeteria line and to model healthy eating behaviors in the cafeteria. Students' positive reactions to the cafeteria foods helped to provide social incentives regarding food choices.

The CATCH Physical Education (PE) component was designed in cooperation with physical education specialists with the goal of increasing the amount of time students spent engaged in moderate to vigorous physical activity during PE class. CATCH PE worked across all three levels of influence. Students learned about the importance of physical activity and built skills to be active during class, focusing on the individual environment. The social environment was influenced by having all students active during class in fun, inclusive games and activities, providing role-modeling, social cues, and reinforcement for being active. The physical environment of PE class was changed by influencing students' accessibility to being active during class. PE teachers modified the content of lessons and how classes were delivered to increase the amount of time that all students were engaged in activity. As an example, elimination games were replaced with games that allowed the entire class to play, and movement activities were incorporated into classroom management time such as taking attendance.

Some CATCH intervention schools also included the CATCH Home Team family component that focused on helping families create more supportive home environments for healthy eating, activity, and avoiding smoking. Home Team materials reinforced the knowledge, attitude, and skill sets learned in the curriculum and encouraged families to offer social support, positive role-modeling, and vicarious learning regarding making health choices about what to eat, how to be active, and not smoking. Families were encouraged to have low-fat foods and snacks available and accessible to children in the home and to provide opportunities for children to be physically active.

At the end of the 3-year intervention, children attending CATCH schools consumed significantly fewer total calories and fewer calories from fat and saturated fat compared with students attending control schools. No statistically significant change was seen in sodium intake or serum cholesterol levels. In addition, students exposed to CATCH PE reported nearly 15 additional minutes of vigorous physical activity per day compared with students in the control schools (Luepker et al., 1996). The school-based Eat Smart and CATCH PE components were successful in significantly reducing the amount of fat and saturated fat offered in school meals and in significantly increasing the amount of active time offered during the PE class, respectively (McKenzie et al., 1996; Osganian et al., 1996).

The CATCH cohort was followed into the eighth grade to determine whether the behavioral changes that were seen at the end of fifth grade had been sustained. Students exposed to CATCH maintained a diet lower in fat and saturated fat intake and continued to report more minutes of vigorous activity compared with those in the control condition (Nader et al., 1999). These findings suggest that the behaviors learned and practiced in elementary school tracked with the children throughout early adolescence. In addition, many of the changes occurring at the schools continued after the research trial was completed and research intervention support withdrawn from the schools (Hoelscher et al., 2004; Lytle et al., 2003; Parcel et al., 2003). Because of its success and its demonstration of long-term change in students and schools exposed to the intervention, CATCH was established as a successful, evidence-based intervention (EBI) and continues to be disseminated nationwide as the Coordinated Approach to Child Health (https://catchinfo.org/). CATCH stands an example of an MLI that was successful in positively influencing children's diet and physical activity, both in the short and long term, as well as an intervention that could be sustained by school systems and disseminated broadly.

DESIGNING MULTILEVEL BEHAVIOR CHANGE INTERVENTIONS: PHASES AND STEPS IN THE PROCESS

Many types of skills and expertise are required to design a community-based intervention, including skills related to understanding health behavior and the process of change, engaging communities, creating interventions strategies that will be meaningful and impactful, and skills related to organizational and project management, communication, evaluation, study design, and data analysis. Designing interventions requires teamwork and may include partners from different institutions representing different communities and stakeholders. Working in teams and with partners to design MLIs is challenging but deeply rewarding.

Once a need for an intervention to promote community health is identified, the team will need to explore if there is an existing intervention that has been shown to be effective in achieving change in a similar behavior with a similar community. The use of an EBI may help ensure that the intervention will result in a positive outcome and may save the team effort, time, and resources. Often, however, EBIs will need to be adapted to better fit the culture of the new community, address differences in resources available, or meet the unique needs of recipients of the intervention including the format of the intervention, language or literacy (Wiltsey Stirman et al., 2019). Chapter 7 of this book suggests ways to use the framework and the intervention design process to adapt EBIs.

Further, there may be no EBIs to use, or the degree of adaptation required to fit the needs of the community is so large as to call into question the integrity— and therefore the effectiveness—of an adapted intervention. In those cases, a team must build the intervention from the ground up. A systematic approach, grounded in science and community-engaged experience, is essential to maximize an intervention's potential to be effective, feasible, and relevant to a community. In addition, a systematic approach enhances what the field can learn about promoting health through behavioral interventions and creating interventions that can be sustained and disseminated.

As a way to guide researchers and practitioners in the process of designing multilevel community interventions, a set of four phases are outlined with steps embedded in each phase. The 12 steps are outlined in Table 1.1. Some intervention teams may want to break down these 12 steps into additional substeps as they see fit to manage their process, but for many teams, these steps will provide sufficient direction for the tasks involved.

TABLE 1.1. Phases and Steps for Designing Multilevel Programs to Promote Community Health

Phase	Steps
Phase 1: Plan	1. Identify a behavior-based community health problem.
	2. Choose the relevant behavioral determinants.
	3. Create a conceptual model.
	4. Review the conceptual model with the evaluation team and community stakeholders.
Phase 2: Create	5. Write the intervention objectives and identify potential intervention components.
	6. Design intervention strategies.
	7. Create a logic model.
	8. Share the logic model with the evaluation team and community stakeholders.
Phase 3: Implement	9. Develop process evaluation measures.
	10. Finalize intervention protocol, training, and materials.
Phase 4: Evaluate	11. Evaluate the effectiveness of the intervention.
	12. Prepare for the next iteration or dissemination of the intervention.

The Plan Phase

The Plan Phase helps the intervention team work through the essential step of identifying or confirming that a health problem of concern to a community has a behavioral basis and is appropriate for a community-based intervention or program. Next, the team will need to examine the known and potential determinants of the behavior in the community of interest; these determinants become the focus of the intervention work. The Plan Phase describes how to use the existing empirical research, health behavior theories that suggest factors that predict behavior, and formative research with the community to identify potential determinants of the health behavior. The primary product of the Plan Phase is a simple conceptual model showing the determinants that the intervention will target. This conceptual model reflects the design framework and also suggests the mechanisms by which behavior change will occur. In Step 4, the intervention team reviews the progress to date and the conceptual model with the evaluation team and community stakeholders, soliciting specific and purposeful feedback on the plan so that any revisions can be made before the Create Phase begins.

There are four steps embedded in the Plan Phase:

1. Identify a behavior-based community health problem.
2. Choose the relevant behavioral determinants.
3. Create a conceptual model.
4. Review the conceptual model with the evaluation team and community stakeholders.

DEFINITIONS AND DISTINCTIONS USED IN THE BOOK

- **Community:** The term *community* is used to describe any group of individuals who have shared interests or concerns. A community may be defined by a geographic area; the places where people work, worship, play, or go to school; or the issues that help give meaning to their identity.

- **Community engagement:** *Community engagement* is the process of working collaboratively with and through groups of people to address issues affecting the well-being of those people (National Center for HIV/AIDS, Viral Hepatitis, STD, and TB Prevention, n.d.).

- **Complex behavior:** *Complex behaviors* are behaviors that are performed regularly, if not daily (e.g., eating, activity). They often require specialized skills or knowledge and are performed in a social context requiring the individual to navigate the social environment at each behavioral decision point. They stand in contrast to intermittent behaviors such as preventive health screenings and dental checkups.

- **Determinant:** The term *determinant* is used throughout this book to describe the factors that are associated with, or predictive of, the health behavior of interest.

- **Intervention or program:** Taplin et al. (2012) defined an *intervention* (or *program*) as a specified strategy or set of strategies, designed to change the knowledge, perceptions, skills and/or behaviors of individuals, groups, or organizations, with the goal of improving health outcomes.

- **Multilevel intervention (MLI):** *MLIs* are interventions designed to influence more than one contextual level, including groups, organizations, and the community (Clauser et al., 2012).

- **Stakeholder:** *Stakeholders* are individuals and organizations that have an interest in or are affected by the intervention and evaluation activities that occur in their community.

- **Theory:** A *theory* is a set of interrelated concepts that attempt to explain and predict events or situations (Glanz et al., 2015b).

- **Theoretical constructs:** The concepts developed or adapted for a particular theory are called *constructs* (Glanz et al., 2015b). For the purpose of designing interventions, constructs from theories represent potential determinants of the behavior.

- **Type I error:** This type of error can occur when evaluating the effectiveness of an intervention if it is deemed to be effective in creating change when the change actually occurred by chance.

- **Type II error:** This type of error can occur when evaluating the effectiveness of an intervention when it is deemed to be ineffective in creating change when actually it was effective.

- **Type III error:** This type of error can occur when evaluating the effectiveness of an intervention when it was not implemented as planned.

The Create Phase

The Create Phase involves taking the determinants identified in the Plan Phase and creating intervention objectives that specify how the determinant will be positively influenced by the intervention. The Create Phase includes choosing the appropriate intervention components to meet those objectives and developing the specific intervention strategies to effect change. In the Create Phase, the theoretical basis that informs the work includes theories that focus on how change happens at the individual level as well as the organizational, community, and policy levels. Finding meaningful ways to involve the community is essential in this phase. The Create Phase includes careful consideration of the resources that will be needed to implement the intervention and document plans and decisions made by creating a logic model. Similar to the Plan Phase, this phase concludes with sharing the intervention plans and logic model with the evaluation team and community stakeholders. This step is repeated because of the importance of circling back to other team members and community stakeholders before implementation activities begin. Keeping community stakeholders involved cannot be viewed as optional or as an afterthought in the design process.

The steps involved in the Create Phase are as follows:

5. Write the intervention objectives and identify potential intervention components.
6. Design intervention strategies.
7. Create a logic model.
8. Share the logic model with the evaluation team and community stakeholders.

The Implement Phase

The Implement Phase starts with considerations of the process evaluation needs. *Process evaluation* is the collection of data for the purpose of understanding how an intervention works. Such information is critically important for explaining the results of an intervention as well as for providing insights for revising, adapting, and disseminating the intervention. In addition, process evaluation is used for quality control, as well as secondary and exploratory analyses. Appropriate process evaluation tools and methods are needed for each intervention component, and this phase describes how those decisions are made. This phase also focuses on the importance of developing intervention protocols, finalizing materials, training interventionists and on-the-ground involvement of intervention staff. This work is essential for ensuring that the intervention is delivered as planned and as a way to document the details of the intervention for the purpose of reporting and sharing the intervention with others.

The steps included in the Implement Phase are as follows:

9. Develop process evaluation measures.
10. Finalize the intervention protocol, training, and materials.

The Evaluate Phase

Designing an intervention to improve community health will involve some type of evaluation to determine whether it is effective in achieving the targeted behavior change. For research studies, that evaluation will be rigorous with strong attention to study design and other considerations to maximize the ability to attribute behavioral change to the intervention. For practitioners, the purpose of the evaluation may be to inform funders or community stakeholders about how the intervention affected the community and to inform future iterations of the program. The Evaluate Phase includes an examination of the intervention's ability to change the behavior of interest as well as the determinants targeted by the intervention. The results of the evaluation are used to modify the intervention for further testing and evaluation, communicate lessons learned to other behavioral scientists or communities, and promote the dissemination of a successful intervention.

The steps included in the Evaluate Phase are as follows:

11. Evaluate the effectiveness of the intervention.
12. Prepare for the next iteration or dissemination of the intervention.

To illustrate the phases and the steps, a hypothetical example of a school-based intervention to reduce middle school students' intake of sugar-sweetened beverages will be used. This program is called Healthy Teens, Healthy Planet and is referred to by this name throughout the book for convenience, although this title is not formally established by the intervention team until Step 6 in the Create Phase (Chapter 4 of this volume) after carefully planning and finalizing the intervention's objectives and strategies.

2

A Practical Guide to Using Health Behavior Theories to Design Multilevel Interventions

Health behavior theories attempt to explain why people engage, or do not engage, in health behaviors and how change occurs. A valuable health behavior theory is useful in predicting a variety of behaviors (from smoking cessation, to medication adherence, to eating behaviors) as well as behaviors across a range of communities (from workers in a rural setting, to youth in elementary schools, to young adults in urban settings). A health behavior theory may also describe how change happens, providing important insights into the process of change. Because change occurs at an individual level and at community, systems, and organizational levels, theories that help describe how individuals, communities, systems, and organizations change are useful.

This chapter begins with a definition of theory and the general purpose of theories. Although theory is useful in all stages of intervention design (Glanz et al., 2015b), its use is particularly important in the Plan and Create Phases. This chapter includes a brief overview of three theories that are useful in the Plan Phase (Chapter 3, this volume) as a way to identify possible determinants of behavior: the health belief model (HBM), the theory of planned behavior (TPB), and the social cognitive theory (SCT). Theories that are useful in the Create Phase (Chapter 4) are those that help describe how change occurs, at an individual level and at a community, systems, or organizational level. This chapter includes examples of five theories that describe how change occurs at the individual and larger system levels, including stages of change, behavior change taxonomy, diffusion of innovation, community engagement, and policy as a prevention strategy. A description of all health behavior theories is beyond the

https://doi.org/10.1037/0000292-003
Designing Interventions to Promote Community Health: A Multilevel, Stepwise Approach, by L. A. Lytle

scope of this book. The text *Health Behavior: Theory, Research, and Practice* (Glanz et al., 2015a) provides an excellent overview of well-researched health behavior theories and is highly recommended as a more in-depth discussion of behavior change theories.

DEFINING THEORY AND THE PURPOSE OF THEORY

Theory is defined as "a set of interrelated constructs, definitions, and propositions that presents a systematic view of phenomena by specifying relations among variables, with the purpose of explaining and predicting phenomena" (Kerlinger, 1986, p. 9). Behavior change theories provide a systematic approach for considering the factors that explain health behavior and suggesting ways to support behavior change (Glanz et al., 2015b). In addition, the use of theory provides a common lexicon for describing the goals of an intervention and designing evaluation efforts—a shared language or set of terms helps enhance the field's ability to share lessons learned and to build upon experiences. Interventions and programs that are developed with some theoretical underpinnings have an increased chance of being effective in changing behavior compared with programs developed based on hunches, intuition, convenience, or past experience (Glanz et al., 2015b).

Useful health behavior theories are both generalizable across a range of behaviors and parsimonious in their approach for explaining behavior and behavior change. Health behavior theories do not have a specific content or topic area, nor are they specific to a certain population group. Their generalizability is an asset as they provide suggestions for answering broad questions such as "Why do people do what they do?" and "How does behavior change happen?"

In the approach used in this book for designing multilevel interventions (MLIs), the goal is not to test theory or develop new theories but rather to use theory to maximize the effectiveness and efficiency of the intervention. Testing or developing new theories is typically the work of researchers. Practitioners are more likely to use theory as a way to ground and inform intervention work. The work of researchers and practitioners should not be seen in opposition but rather as a dialogue that enriches and strengthens the work of each group and endeavors to enhance population health.

Theory, research, and practice merge when theories are applied in real-world contexts and settings, as when designing community-based interventions. The relationship between theory, research, and practice is cyclical and involves both inductive and deductive reasoning. The cycle begins when observations about a phenomenon are generated from real-life experiences in real-world settings and organized in a way to suggest patterns (inductive reasoning). That organization includes coming up with a common lexicon for naming predictive factors or determinants and identifying potential relations among determinants to explain the phenomena of interest. This process leads to a theory to be evaluated through research with a goal of determining how useful the theory is in explaining and predicting similar phenomena in other settings and populations (deductive reasoning). The findings of that research stimulate more research, and when the theory's utility in explaining the phenomenon has been established, those findings are used by practitioners to help design interventions to promote community health.

THEORIES USEFUL IN THE PLAN PHASE: UNDERSTANDING THE DETERMINANTS OF BEHAVIOR

The primary goals of the Plan Phase are to understand the factors, or determinants, that are associated with or predictive of the behavior of interest in the community and to choose a set of determinants as the focus of the intervention. In the Plan Phase (Chapter 3), the intervention team learns how to identify potential behavioral determinants by (a) examining the empirical research, (b) conducting qualitative evaluation with the community of interest, and (c) choosing determinants or constructs from existing behavior change theories. The behavior change theories that have stood the test of time are those that have identified a set of constructs that have reliably been shown to predict or explain a variety of health behaviors across a range of populations and settings. Constructs are the primary building blocks or elements of a specific theory. The presentation of those constructs and how they relate to each other and to outcomes as a way to explain phenomena is the definition of theory (Glanz et al., 2015b). When designing community-based interventions, constructs from across a wide range of behavioral theories are considered as the potential determinants of behavior, with the intervention focusing on how to positively impact those constructs or determinants.

A brief introduction to three of the most commonly used theories that describe the determinants associated with or predictive of a behavior of interest follows, including the HBM (Becker, 1974), the TPB/integrated behavioral model (Ajzen, 1991; Montano & Kasprzyk, 2015), and SCT (Bandura, 1986).

The Health Belief Model

The HBM was developed in the 1950s by social psychologists trying to explain why people were not taking advantage of screening for tuberculosis. Despite the convenience of screening vans sent into communities, participation in screening was low, increasing the chance of community-wide infection. The model developers used a value–expectancy approach to posit why people would engage in screening behavior. This approach begins with an assumption that behavior is a function of the degree to which an individual values an outcome and their assessment of the probability or expectation that a defined behavior will result in a desired outcome. In short, value represents how important it is to the individual to avoid illness or promote wellness, while expectancy represents one's expectation that the behavior may prevent or ameliorate risk. The HBM focuses on understanding how people's attitudes regarding individual-level risk and the costs and benefits of changing their behavior to reduce that risk will influence their health behavior.

There are six main constructs in the HBM (Skinner et al., 2015):

- **Perceived susceptibility:** Beliefs about the likelihood of getting a disease or condition.

- **Perceived severity:** Beliefs about the seriousness of contracting an illness or condition. Perceptions of severity include beliefs about the physical and social consequences of the illness or condition.

- **Perceived benefits:** Beliefs about the positive aspects of adopting the preventive or health promotive behavior. These include personal health, social and economic benefits.

- **Perceived barriers:** Beliefs about the obstacles to performing the preventive behavior and the negative aspects of adopting the behavior. These barriers including inconvenience, fear, and cost, including economic and social costs.

- **Cues to action:** Internal or external factors that could trigger the preventive behavior. The cue could be internal (e.g., feeling pain or discomfort in the body) or external (e.g., getting a reminder for an upcoming medical appointment).

- **Self-efficacy:** Beliefs that one can perform the recommended behavior.

Perceptions of susceptibility and severity represent the individual's assessment of the degree of threat that they are exposing themselves to by not enacting a risk-reducing or health-promotive behavior. Consider a woman deciding whether she should have mammography screening for the detection of breast cancer. Perceived susceptibility and severity might be represented as the woman ponders, "How likely is it that I might have breast cancer? Does breast cancer run in my family? If I do have breast cancer, how bad (severe) would it be? Is it a disease that I can live with without having a large impact on my quality of life?" The greater the estimate of threat, the greater is one's estimate of the potential value, or importance, of getting screened. If a person does not perceive any threat, it is unlikely that they will engage in the behavior (getting screened).

Perceptions of benefits and barriers represent weighing the benefits of engaging in the recommended behavior against the barriers or costs of the behavior. Again, using the mammography screening example, the woman might weigh her perceptions of benefits by considering, "If I'm screened for breast cancer and found not to have it, I will feel so relieved. If I get a mammogram and they find something, it will be much better to find out now and begin treatment at an early stage." Barriers that might be considered include "If I find out I have cancer, how will I continue to work and support my family? Are mammograms safe? Will I feel uncomfortable getting a mammogram?" People are more likely to engage in a behavior if they believe that the benefits outweigh the barriers. Cues to action in this example might include a lump detected during a breast self-exam, learning that a friend was diagnosed with breast cancer, or getting a text reminder from a clinic that it is time for one's annual mammogram. The construct of self-efficacy originated in the SCT and was added to the HBM to help explain complex behaviors, such as eating, activity, or smoking cessation, that require some skill set to accomplish and maintain the behavior over time. That skill set may include motivational or self-regulation skills, social or communication skills, or behavioral "how-to" skills. Self-efficacy does not apply well to simple, one-time, or intermittent behaviors, such as screening, vaccination, or scheduling annual checkups (Weinstein, 2007).

The HBM is a relatively simple theory that focuses on factors related to decision making. Originally the theory focused on people's perceptions of their risk and perceptions of benefits and barriers associated with the behavior; perceptions represent determinants from the individual environment. Over time, however, the theory has evolved to include consideration of actual barriers and benefits that exist in individuals' social and physical environments. As an example, an intervention drawing on the HBM may include patient navigators as social support for women making decisions about mammography screening. Likewise, a decision about getting a mammogram will include consideration of the availability of mammography screening in one's community as well as costs associated with screening. Perceptions remain extremely important, particularly for susceptibility and severity. Risk denial is a strong human tendency, and one's actual risk (based on patient history, behaviors, and biomarkers) might be very different from their perceived risk.

INSIGHTS FOR INTERVENTIONISTS: THE UTILITY OF THE HBM FOR IDENTIFYING DETERMINANTS OF BEHAVIOR

For interventionists looking for possible determinants to include in their intervention planning, the HBM suggests that understanding people's perceptions of risk is important; intervention efforts may need to focus on increasing one's awareness of their risk through education or counseling. Likewise, if individuals' perceptions of the benefits and barriers related to a behavior have a negative impact on their decision to change, those determinants may be important to include in the intervention planning, with a goal of shifting perceptions either through persuasion, providing skill-building activities to increase self-efficacy, or by working to remove actual barriers in the social and physical environment. Providing tangible benefits for behavior may be important in the early stages of behavior change, but eventually benefits of the behavior need to be internalized to promote lasting change. Cues to action can be a useful determinant to consider and can include traditional methods such as reminder calls, the use of social media to cue behavior, or may include a more stealth approach to instigate behavior.

The Theory of Planned Behavior

The TPB is another theory that focuses on individual-level factors and their relationship to each other and a behavioral outcome. The TPB adds intention, subjective norm, and perceived control to the attitudes included in the HBM as important predictors or correlates of behavior (Montano & Kasprzyk, 2015). The main constructs from the TPB are as follows.

- **Behavioral intention:** Perceived likelihood of performing the behavior.

- **Attitude:** Overall evaluation of the behavior; belief that behavioral performance is associated with certain outcomes and the values attached to those outcomes.

- **Subjective norm:** Belief about whether most people approve or disapprove of the behavior.

- **Perceived control:** Belief about how much control the individual has to enact the behavior.

The TPB posits that intention is the best predictor of actual behavior because it represents that a decision has been made to engage in the behavior. For example, "I intend to call the clinic and schedule my mammogram" indicates that the woman has considered all the factors related to screening and has decided that she will be screened. The association between intention and behavior is variable, however. Motivations may lag and barriers emerge between the time that the decision is made and the behavioral opportunity. As an example, the woman intending to get a mammogram misses her appointment when she is unable to find transportation to the clinic.

The constructs representing attitudes in the TPB include the constructs used in the HBM, including perceived susceptibility, severity, benefits, and barriers (both the TPB and the HBM are value–expectancy models) as well as a construct representing overall evaluation of the behavior. For example, an attitude toward screening might include one's overall evaluation of screening: "Is screening a wise or foolish thing to do?" "Is screening a good or bad thing to do?"

The TPB advances the HBM by adding the constructs of subjective norm and perceived control. Subjective norm represents one's belief regarding whether other people who are important to them approve or disapprove of the behavior and an assessment of one's motivation to comply with other's expectations. Subjective norm is part of the individual environment because it represents people's *perceptions* of what they think that others want them to do and may or may not reflect reality. As an example, a woman may think that her family would disapprove of her getting a mammogram because of cultural beliefs about modesty, but that may not reflect her family members' actual beliefs. Motivation to comply is also part of subjective norm. Even if one's family does not support a woman's decision to get a mammogram, she may believe that it is important and decide to get a mammogram irrespective of their beliefs.

The construct of perceived control is similar to the construct of self-efficacy (Fishbein & Ajzen, 2010). However, self-efficacy is more of a psychological construct representing an estimation of one's confidence in being able to perform the behavior, whereas perceived control also addresses that behavior is not always volitional; sometimes things outside the control of the individual prevent behavior. Likewise, perceived control is similar to perceived barriers from the HBM because it refers to one's assessment of the presence or absence of barriers to behavioral performance as well as one's perceived power to overcome barriers. Perceived control points to the importance of the physical environment in shaping behavior, as people's sense of control will be diminished if opportunity to enact a behavior is not available. As with the HBM, the TPB's original focus was on the individual environment as beliefs or perceptions were identified in the theory's constructs as predicting intention to behave and behavior. Over time, research and intervention work has expanded these constructs to include elements of the social and physical environment that influence one's volitional control over their behavior as well as their beliefs and perceptions. The TPB points to the importance of changing perceptions but also to changing the realities in the social and physical environment that feed those perceptions.

INSIGHTS FOR INTERVENTIONISTS: THE UTILITY OF THE TPB FOR IDENTIFYING DETERMINANTS OF BEHAVIOR

For interventionists looking for possible determinants to include in their intervention planning, the TPB suggests that beyond the attitudes identified in the HBM, people's perceptions about how others view their behavior is an important predictor of behavior. This influence is strongest from people who are in our closest social networks, including our family, friends, and others who care about us. It is important for interventionists to understand who in one's social network holds the greatest influence for the behavior in question because those individuals or groups will likely garner the most influence. Subjective norm is a determinant that fits in the individual environment because it reflects one's perceptions of social influence. One's perceived control of a situation may include a consideration of one's confidence in their ability to behave in a certain way (self-efficacy) but may also represent a consideration of the actual obstacles to the behavior. The construct of perceived control can remind interventionists to look for real and perceived barriers in one's social or physical environment that would impede health behavior and apply intervention strategies to reduce those barriers.

The Social Cognitive Theory

The SCT is one of the most widely applied models of health behavior and is particularly well suited for complex behaviors and MLIs. Complex behaviors are those that must be performed regularly, if not daily, requiring active decision making until a behavioral pattern forms. Complex behaviors often require some specialized knowledge or skills to perform the behavior and typically are performed within a social context requiring the individual to navigate the social environment at each decision point. Examples of complex behaviors include eating, physical activity and sedentary behaviors, sexual behaviors, sleep, and alcohol and tobacco use. They stand in contrast to intermittent behaviors, such as screening behaviors, vaccinations, and regular dental and medical checkups (Weinstein, 2007).

Key to the SCT is the concept of *reciprocal determinism*, a dynamic model of causation where supporting cognitive influences, behavioral factors, and the physical and social environment interact to explain human behavior (Kelder et al., 2015). Constructs from the SCT are organized by the following three elements of reciprocal determinism:

- Cognitive influences on behavior

  - Self-efficacy: A person's confidence in their ability to perform a behavior.

  - Outcome expectations: Judgments about the likely consequences of actions.

  - Knowledge: An understanding of the health risks and benefits of health practices and information necessary to perform a behavior.

- Social and physical environmental influences on behavior

  - Observational learning: Learning that occurs by observing the behaviors of others and witnessing the consequences of their behaviors (also referred to as vicarious learning).

  - Normative beliefs: Cultural norms and beliefs about the social acceptability and perceived prevalence of a behavior.

  - Social support: Real and perceived encouragement and support a person receives from their social networks.

  - Barriers and opportunities: Attributes of the social or physical environment that make behaviors more difficult or easier to perform.

- Supporting behavioral factors

  - Intentions: Expression of a goal or intention to add new behaviors or modify existing behaviors.

  - Behavioral skills: The abilities needed to successfully perform a behavior.

  - Reinforcement and punishment: The provision or removal of rewards or punishments for particular behaviors.

The SCT suggests determinants that are important for both initiating a behavior and maintaining a behavior over time. Self-efficacy is one of the most robust constructs from the SCT and represents one's confidence in their ability to perform a behavior. It includes confidence in being able to perform skills specific to the behavior, including cognitive skills ("Can I learn how to understand food labels so that I can make good choices at the grocery store?"), social skills ("Can I negotiate rules around noise and light with my roommates to create a better sleep environment at our apartment?"), and behavioral skills ("Can I build cooking skills to prepare healthy meals for my family?"). Self-efficacy also includes one's confidence in their ability to resist urges that threaten the long-term viability of the behavior change ("Will I be able to resist the urge to smoke when I am stressed?"). Some level of confidence (self-efficacy) is necessary for an individual to consider attempting a new behavior and efficacy-enhancing skills are useful in maintaining behavior.

Outcome expectations refer to one's assessment of how likely a behavior will result in a desired outcome and includes physical, social, and self-evaluative consequences; as a construct, it is similar to perceived benefits and barriers from other value–expectancy theories. Imagine that a young adult wants to increase his levels of physical activity to lose weight and feel more energetic. When considering outcome expectations, he may wonder, "If I am more active, will I actually lose weight and feel more energetic?" (physical consequences); "Will my friends tease me?" (social consequences); and "Will I be able to stick with it this time?" (self-evaluation). The construct of knowledge is often assumed in behavioral theories. Knowledge includes *why* and *what* knowledge ("Why is it important for me to be more active? What are the recommended minutes of physical activity for young adults?") as well as *how* knowledge ("How do I begin to exercise safely so I don't get hurt? How do I build an exercise routine that will provide cardiovascular benefits as well as strength and flexibility?"). Decades of research in health education and behavior have demonstrated that knowledge is a necessary but not sufficient condition for behavior change.

Observational learning is a key element of the social environment and refers to what people learn about how to behave from observing others' behavior, as well as the consequences (negative and positive) to expect from enacting the behavior. Vicarious learning is another term for observational learning. One's exposure to "actors" in one's environment provides important information to an individual about what to expect should they change their behavior. Importantly, observational learning can occur without the actors in the environment realizing that their behavior is being observed or is at all influential. As an example, a young adult who is considering increasing activity levels may learn about how easy, or difficult, being more active is by observing a friend or colleague's experience. Likewise, they may be able to anticipate rewards if they see the benefits accrued (i.e., weight loss, stress relief, support from others) by that friend or colleague. The term *role-modeling* is frequently used interchangeably with *observational learning* and *vicarious learning* but often suggests a more deliberate approach to observational learning in which individuals are designated as "role models" for others and are aware that they are being observed.

Observational learning is related to normative beliefs which are formed by watching one's social group and assessing how common or unusual a behavior is. Normative beliefs reflect what is socially and culturally acceptable to a group. The sentiment that "none of my friends exercise because they are all too busy" sets up a normative belief that would hinder the initiation of an exercise program.

Social support represents perceptions of support (from the individual environment) and actual support received (from the social environment). On the perception side, a young adult may believe "If I'm going to start exercising, I will need to do it on my own; none of my friends will want to exercise with me," and this perception may be accurate, or not. Actual social support is typically classified into four categories: emotional support (providing care and companionship), esteem support (validating beliefs and emotions), informational support (providing information or advice), and instrumental or tangible support (providing help with a task or offering financial support; Holt-Lunstad & Uchino, 2015). Using the physical activity example, finding a coach at the local gym may provide social support across all of these categories.

Barriers and opportunities include one's perceptions about how attributes of the social and physical environments will impact their change attempt as well as real barriers that exist in those environments. In the exercise example, barriers might include perceptions that it is not safe to walk or run in one's neighborhood as well as real barriers in the physical environment that make being active outside difficult, such as lack of street lighting and sidewalks.

Finally, the constructs related to behavioral factors include intention (similar to the TPB) and suggest that behavior change begins with a decision to change. Other important constructs include behavioral skills, referring specifically to having the abilities to enact the behavior, and self-regulation skills, such as knowing how to self-monitor one's behaviors, set goals, and identify ways to reinforce positive behavior and make corrections when behavior attempts lapse. For the young adult trying to increase his level of physical activity, this may include teaching him how to monitor specific aspects of his behavior (i.e., the number of steps he takes in a day or the number of minutes spent daily in moderate to vigorous physical activity), how to set realistic goals to increase his activity over time, and how to deal with setbacks and lapses. Finally, the SCT specifically addresses how reinforcement and punishment may be factors that predict behavior. Our earliest stimulus–response theories (Skinner, 1938; Watson, 1925) stressed the importance of behavioral cues (antecedents) and reinforcements (consequences) in eliciting a reflexive behavioral response that did not involve any decision making. Although the SCT recognizes the importance of cognition and active decision making, the power of reinforcements (even those that are not cognitively recognized) in eliciting and sustaining behavior is well established. For community-based MLIs, punishments are rarely used, but finding ways to reinforce behaviors with both tangible

INSIGHTS FOR INTERVENTIONISTS: THE UTILITY OF THE SCT FOR IDENTIFYING DETERMINANTS OF BEHAVIOR

The SCT provides interventionists with a rich source of potential determinants. SCT suggests that increasing one's self-efficacy is an essential step toward behavior change. Specific intervention strategies can be used to increase self-efficacy such as providing opportunities for incremental behavior change and reinforcement. The SCT also stresses that both knowledge about the behavior and skills to accomplish the behavior are essential. Building skills to enhance behavioral capacity such as self-regulation, self-monitoring, and goal setting can be powerful intervention strategies, especially for complex behaviors. Importantly, SCT cues the interventionist to examine potential determinants in the social environment including the use of observational learning, role models, and social support to support behavior change.

assets (i.e., money) and intangible assets (i.e., praise) are associated with behavior change.

THEORIES USEFUL IN THE CREATE PHASE: UNDERSTANDING THE PROCESS OF CHANGE

The primary goal of the Create Phase (Chapter 4) is to determine how the intervention will be created to effect change. Just as there are behavioral theories that help identify the determinants to be changed, there are theories that are helpful in understanding the process of change. Two theories that examine how change occurs at the individual level are briefly reviewed here, including the transtheoretical model (TTM; Prochaska et al., 2015) and the use of a behavior change taxonomy (Michie et al., 2013). In examining how change occurs at a systems level, I review diffusion of innovation (Rogers, 2003, Chapter 1), community change approaches through community engagement (Wallerstein et al., 2015), and the multiple streams framework for policy change (Kingdon, 2011).

The Transtheoretical Model/Stages of Change: How Change Happens in Individuals

The TTM represents the integration of concepts from more than 300 theories from psychotherapy and includes four sets of constructs to explain how change occurs: stages of change, processes of change, decisional balance, and self-efficacy (Prochaska et al., 2015).

Stages of change suggests that change proceeds through six distinct phases. These phases often occur in a nonlinear manner with people moving back and forward between stages. The six stages identified are as follows:

- **Precontemplation:** At this stage, the individual has no intention of changing their behavior in the next 6 months. They may be in this stage because they are not aware of or concerned about the risks associated with their behavior or they may have tried to change in the past, failed, and are at a point where they are not interested in trying to change. People in this stage will need to be motivated to consider changing their behavior.

- **Contemplation:** At this stage the individual intends to change their behavior in the next 6 months. They are considering the pros and cons of behavior change but are still in the process of making up their minds about actually trying to change their behavior. These people might need encouragement or information on how to initiate change.

- **Preparation:** At this stage, individuals intend to act soon, as early as in the next month. They may have already taken some steps toward change—for example, telling a partner of their intent to change a behavior or signing up for a class to help with the change. People in this stage of change need encouragement and reinforcement and may need help in skill-building or information-seeking related to change.

- **Action:** Individuals in the action stage have taken concrete steps in the past 6 months to change a behavior. They need support, encouragement, and reminders that change is difficult and that a slip does not mean that they have failed; they need to be encouraged to continue to learn from the process and to keep trying.

- **Maintenance:** Individuals in maintenance have made specific, demonstrable changes in their behavior and are working to prevent relapse. This maintenance phase may last between 6 months to 5 years as individuals continue to meet the challenges of avoiding relapse. Individuals who reach this phase may need very little support from an interventionist until some stress occurs and leads to a slip in behavior. Then, the interventionist's role is to help the individual problem solve how to better handle the next slip and to continue to reinforce that they are making important changes.

- **Termination:** This is the final phase where the previous health behavior is completely eliminated from their behavioral repertoire and the individual feels no temptation to relapse. The interventionist's job is done!

Another major set of constructs from the TTM are the processes of change (Prochaska et al., 2015). The following processes are believed to be helpful in moving people through stages:

- **Consciousness raising:** Increasing awareness of the causes and consequences of the problem behavior and the benefits of change.

- **Dramatic relief:** Increasing negative or positive emotions to motivate change. The use of fear arousal is an example of dramatic relief.

- **Self-evaluation:** Reassessing one's self-image relative to changing a behavior.

- **Environmental reevaluation:** Increasing awareness of how one's behavior affects one's social environment—for example, the impact of smoking on one's family, both from passive smoking as well as role modeling for children in the family.

- **Self-liberation:** Working to instill the belief that one can change, building one's self-efficacy about their ability to change.

- **Helping relationships:** Encouraging the development and nurturing of a positive social network that supports healthy behavior change.

- **Social liberation:** Increasing healthy behavioral options in one's social or physical environment.

- **Counterconditioning:** Changing the cues in one's social or physical environment to help make the healthy choice the easy choice.

- **Stimulus control:** Removing behavioral cues for less healthy habits and adding cues for healthier alternatives.

- **Reinforcement management:** Encouraging self-reinforcement or reinforcement from others for making healthy behavioral choices.

Certain processes are believed to be important at specific stages. For individuals who are in the precontemplation or contemplation stages, intervention strategies will need to focus on raising awareness of why change is important and how change would benefit the individual (consciousness raising). Motivation is also essential in these early stages and may involve using fear arousal or finding inspirational stories from others (dramatic relief). In these early stages, people can also be motivated to change by increasing their awareness of how their behavior is affecting others (environmental evaluation). For those moving into the preparation stage, self-evaluation strategies may be helpful because they are encouraged to imagine how they will feel (physically, socially, and emotionally) when they succeed at changing the behavior. As they move into the action phase, individuals will need to learn how to make small changes that will build their confidence and resolve and help them persevere when it becomes difficult to change their habits (building self-efficacy). As part of both the action and maintenance phases, they will need to learn how to eliminate or manage cues in the environment that encourage their old behavior while creating new environmental cues for the new behavior (stimulus control) and how reinforce themselves for positive behavior changes (reinforcement management). Those in the action stage and maintenance phases will need social and emotional support to persist, feedback on their accomplishments, and to replace old behaviors with healthier behaviors (helping relationships and counterconditioning).

INSIGHTS FOR INTERVENTIONISTS: THE UTILITY OF THE TTM/STAGES OF CHANGE FOR EXAMINING HOW CHANGE HAPPENS IN INDIVIDUALS

For the purpose of designing interventions, the important ideas that the TTM brings are that (a) change happens in stages, (b) different processes of change may be useful in moving individuals from one stage to the next, and (c) change is facilitated when the person can come to evaluate the benefits of change as exceeding the barriers to change and through activities that help build the individual's self-confidence in their ability to change. The importance of knowing an individual's stage of behavior change and providing tailored intervention strategies are key elements for interventionists to consider.

The last two constructs in the TTM are familiar from the health behavior theories previously described as part of the Plan Phase. Decisional balance involves encouraging change by having one consider the benefits of changing versus the costs of changing (similar to the benefits and barriers constructs from the HBM; Becker, 1974). The construct of self-efficacy comes from the SCT (Bandura, 1986) and refers to one's confidence in their ability to enact the behavior across a variety of situations.

TTM approaches have been used to change a variety of health behaviors, including smoking, dietary behaviors, exercise, sexual behaviors, and medication adherence. The most common application of the TTM is the use of interventionist-delivered change strategies tailored to individuals. The process begins by staging an individual using a set of questions to identify the stage of change where the individual is beginning their behavior change attempt. Over a period of time, the interventionist provides tailored messages (delivered in person or through print or electronic messaging) to help move the individual toward the action and maintenance phases. (Noar et al., 2007). The TTM has also been used to effect change at the group level (e.g., changing the diet behaviors of children in schools or church congregations) but with mixed success (Aveyard et al., 1999). It is more difficult to design such tailored strategies for groups because individuals within a group will start at different stages of change, and their progress through the stages will vary. In addition, the effectiveness of the TTM appears to vary by how many of the TTM constructs were used in the intervention (Spencer et al., 2002).

Behavior Change Techniques and Taxonomy: How Change Happens in Individuals

Like the TTM, the work on identifying behavior change techniques (BCTs) through the use of a behavior change taxonomy has its roots in clinical psychology. Its focus is on understanding and labeling the active ingredients in complex interventions designed to change behavior.

Interventions to change behavior oftentimes use many different approaches or techniques to reach the behavioral goal. For example, a weight-loss intervention may include self-monitoring, setting goals, limiting cues to overeating, asking for social support, and building new skills related to food preparation. These techniques may be used over a period of time in different combinations, with different emphases and intensities, but all of the activities combined are evaluated as a single entity representing the "intervention." Sometimes this compilation of intervention activities is called the intervention "black box" (Pearson et al., 2001). The details of the intervention strategies used are lost when the effectiveness of the intervention is evaluated; we may know that "the intervention" was or was not successful in changing behavior, but we know very little else about how the intervention worked or if some aspects of the intervention were more important than others.

The lack of standardization in the language used to describe intervention strategies also limits our ability to learn from other interventions. For example, having intervention participants record their behavior might be called "self-diaries" by one group, "behavioral logs" by another, and "self-monitoring" by yet another group. The absence of a common lexicon to describe intervention strategies limits our ability to compare the effectiveness of interventions, understand the content and mechanism of the interventions, and replicate and implement those interventions found to be successful.

In an attempt to advance the ability to describe, design, and implement effective behavior change interventions, Michie and colleagues (2013) advocated for deconstructing complex interventions into their active ingredients; they called these active ingredients BCTs and defined them as an "observable, replicable and irreducible component of an intervention designed to alter or redirect causal processes that regulate behavior" (p. 82). Michie et al. saw the identification and compilation of BCTs as an aid to intervention development and referred to this compilation of BCTs (with clear labels, definitions, and examples) as a taxonomy.

The process of building the taxonomy involved engaging international behavior change experts, primarily psychologists, in a multistaged consensus process to identify and name discrete BCTs used in interventions (Michie et al., 2013). The experts identified 93 unique BCTs within 16 clusters or domains, with domains representing a higher-level category of a group of BCTs. Table 2.1 lists the 16 domains identified through this process, the total numbers of BCTs identified for each domain, and an example of two BCTs within each domain. As an example, nine BCTs were identified representing intervention strategies around a domain labeled "Goals and Planning." One of the BCTs within the domain is goal setting related to the desired behavioral outcome (i.e., "I will practice 5 minutes of mindful meditation at least 5 days a week"), while another BCT within this domain involves problem-solving activities (e.g., "Make a list of three things that make it difficult for you to practice mindful meditation. Now, come up with a strategy for how you will eliminate each barrier"). (For a

TABLE 2.1. Behavior Change Domains and Examples of Behavior Change Techniques (BCTs) Within Each Domain

Domain	Sample BCTs
Goals and Planning (Nine BCTs)	**Goal setting (behavior):** Set or agree on a goal defined in terms of the behavior to be achieved.
	Problem solving: Analyze factors influencing the behavior and generate or select strategies that include overcoming barriers and/or increasing facilitators.
Feedback and Monitoring (Seven BCTs)	**Self-monitoring of behavior:** Establish a method for the person to monitor and record their behavior(s) as part of a behavior change strategy.
	Feedback on outcome of the behavior: Monitor and provide feedback on the outcome of performance of the behavior.
Social Support (Three BCTs)	**Social support, practical:** Advise on, arrange, or provide practical help for performance of the behavior.
	Social support, emotional: Advise on, arrange, or provide emotional support for performance of the behavior.
Shaping Knowledge (Four BCTs)	**Instruction on how to perform a behavior:** Advise or agree on how to perform the behavior (includes skills training).
	Information about antecedents: Provide information about antecedents that reliably predict performance of the behavior.
Natural Consequences (Six BCTs)	**Monitoring of emotional consequences:** Prompt assessment of feelings after attempts at performing the behavior.
	Anticipated regret: Induce or raise awareness of expectations of future regret about performance of the unwanted behavior.
Comparison of Behavior (Three BCTs)	**Social comparison:** Draw attention to others' performance to allow comparison with the person's own performance.
	Information about others' approval: Provide information about what other people think about the behavior. The information clarifies whether others will like, approve, or disapprove of what the person is doing or will do.
Associations (Eight BCTs)	**Prompts/cues:** Introduce or define environmental or social stimulus with the purpose of prompting or cueing the behavior. The prompt or cue would normally occur at the time or place of performance.
	Remove access to the reward: Advise or arrange for the person to be separated from situations in which unwanted behavior can be rewarded to reduce the behavior.
Repetition and Substitution (Seven BCTs)	**Behavioral practice/rehearsal:** Prompt practice or rehearsal of the performance of the behavior one or more times in a context or at a time when the performance may not be necessary to increase habit and skill.
	Graded tasks: Set easy-to-perform tasks, making them increasingly difficult, but achievable, until the behavior is performed.
Comparison of Outcomes (Three BCTs)	**Credible source:** Present verbal or visual communication from a credible source in favor of or against the behavior.
	Comparative imagining of future outcomes: Prompt or advise the imagining and comparing of future outcomes of changed versus unchanged behavior.

TABLE 2.1. Behavior Change Domains and Examples of Behavior Change Techniques (BCTs) Within Each Domain (*Continued*)

Domain	Sample BCTs
Reward and Threat (11 BCTs)	**Material incentive:** Inform that money, vouchers, or other valued objects will be delivered if and only if there has been effort and/or progress in performing the behavior.
	Self-reward: Prompt self-praise or self-reward if and only if there has been effort or progress in performing the behavior.
Regulation (Four BCTs)	**Pharmacological support:** Provide, or encourage the use of or adherence to, drugs to facilitate behavior change.
	Reduce negative emotions: Advise on ways of reducing negative emotions to facilitate performance of the behavior (includes stress management).
Antecedents (Six BCTs)	**Restructuring the physical environment:** Change or advise to change the physical environment to facilitate performance of the wanted behavior or create barriers to the unwanted behavior.
	Adding objects to the environment: Add objects to the environment to facilitate the performance of the behavior.
Identity (Five BCTs)	**Identification of self as role model:** Inform that one's own behavior may be an example to others.
	Incompatible beliefs: Draw attention to discrepancies between current or past behavior and self-image to create discomfort (includes "cognitive dissonance").
Scheduled Consequences (10 BCTs)	**Behavior cost:** Arrange for withdrawal of something valued if (and only if) an unwanted behavior is performed.
	Reward approximation: Arrange for rewards following any approximation to the target behavior, gradually rewarding only performance closer to the wanted behavior (includes shaping).
Self-Belief (Four BCTs)	**Verbal persuasion about capability:** Tell the person that they can successfully perform the wanted behavior, arguing against self-doubts and asserting that they can and will succeed.
	Self-talk: Prompt positive self-talk (aloud or silently) before and during the behavior.
Covert Learning (Three BCTs)	**Imaginary reward:** Advise to imagine performing the wanted behavior in a real-life situation followed by imagining a pleasant consequence.
	Vicarious consequences: Prompt observation of the consequences (including rewards and punishments) for others when they perform the behavior.

Note. The BCT definitions are reproduced from the BCT-Taxonomy training website (https://www. bct-taxonomy.com/).

INSIGHTS FOR INTERVENTIONISTS: THE UTILITY OF THE BEHAVIOR CHANGE TAXONOMY FOR EXAMINING HOW CHANGE HAPPENS IN INDIVIDUALS

For the purpose of designing interventions, the behavior change taxonomy suggests specific behavior change techniques that can be used in creating intervention approaches and strategies. Using the 16 domains identified, interventionists can consider which types of intervention approaches are needed. For example, does this community need to be more conscious of their behavior? If so, consider BCTs from the domain of Feedback and Monitoring. Would social support increase the chances that behavior change could occur? If so, consider behavior change techniques from the domain of Social Support. It is unlikely that all domains will be used in planning an intervention. Choices will be made during the Plan Phase based on information gleaned about the community and how they experience the behavior.

complete listing and description of the 93 BCTs, as well as training on coding interventions using the taxonomy, see the BCT taxonomy training website: https://www.bct-taxonomy.com/.) The use of a behavior change taxonomy has grown in popularity in the past decade and has been used internationally to describe interventions and synthesize evidence. To date, a post hoc approach has been used in which interventions are deconstructed into their component BCTs after the intervention has already been developed. The BCT taxonomy training website includes a compendium of articles that have examined BCTs across interventions.

Diffusion of Innovation: How Change Happens in Organizations and Communities

Diffusion of innovation (DOI) was one of the first theories developed to examine how change happens in systems or organizations. DOI was originally conceived as an approach to understand how agricultural innovations (e.g., irrigation practices, seed use) spread across farmers in the midwestern United States. It considered both the types of individuals who were most likely to be the early adopters of new innovations and how the characteristics of innovations influenced the rate in which they were adopted (Rogers, 2003, Chapter 1). Innovation refers to any idea, practice, or object that is perceived as new by an individual or other units of adoption, such as a worksite, social group, or organization (Brownson et al., 2015). A change in social norms about drinking and driving would represent an *idea* as an innovation, while adopting a policy to restrict smoking at a worksite would be an innovation related to *practice*. Encouraging the use of compostable dishware for takeout restaurants represents an innovation as an *object*.

Unique to DOI is the key premise that some innovations diffuse quickly and widely, while others are abandoned after a relatively short trial. Insights into the factors that may inhibit or facilitate the adoption of an innovation are especially useful for interventionists (Brownson et al., 2015). These insights include a consideration of the following factors:

- **Perceptions of cost:** Adoption may be hampered if key decision makers believe that the cost of adopting and implementing the innovation is not worth the benefit expected. These costs may include time, effort, and resources.

- **Compatibility:** Adoption may be hampered if the innovation requires significant change in how things are currently done and disruption to the existing routine.

- **Observability:** Adoption may be hampered if key decision makers believe that the benefits of the outcome will not be recognized or observed by key stakeholders. Alternatively, if the innovation involves a great deal of risk and the innovation fails, observability may refer to the risk of having the failure observable to stakeholders.

- **Trialability:** Adoption may be enhanced if the innovation can be phased in and piloted before full adoption is required.

- **Relative advantage:** Adoption may be enhanced to the degree that key decision makers believe that the innovation will be better than what it will displace.

- **Simplicity:** Adoption may be enhanced when the changes involved with the innovation are easy to understand and to implement.

Another important premise of DOI is that those individuals who are comfortable with risk taking and eager to find better ways to improve places, situations, or things (called *innovators* or *early adopters*) are key to the uptake and spread of the innovation. For interventionists planning strategies for change, identifying these innovators may be key in promoting the adoption and the spread of the innovation. These innovators are often also opinion leaders of a group and can act as important role models, showing others still considering change how challenges were overcome and the benefits that the new innovation has brought to them or their organization.

Finally, DOI is similar to the TTM in that it uses a stage-ordered process to describe how innovations are adopted. The first stage of the process is awareness when an individual or organizational unit is exposed to the innovation and begins to see how the innovation may function and be useful to solve a problem. The second stage is persuasion where an evaluation of the innovation is formed (either positive or negative) about adopting the innovation. The next stage is the decision stage, during which activities that will lead to either adopting or rejecting an innovation occur. Implementation is the next stage, in which the innovation is put in place. The staging ends with confirmation where the individual or organizational unit seeks reinforcement for a decision made. The similarities with the TTM/stages of change are shown in Table 2.2.

APPLYING DIFFUSION OF INNOVATION CONCEPTS

Example A: Changing Menu Options at a University Dining Hall

A university dining service wants to encourage students to choose plant-based entrée options by making more vegan entrée options available. The rationale for this change is to improve the nutritional health of students as well as reduce the negative impact of a meat-based diet on planetary health. Because of restricted space on the serving lines, this change will require offering fewer meat-based entrée options. In considering this change (or innovation), the administrative and food service staff will need to think about the following:

The cost of the change: How long will it take to identify and evaluate suitable plant-based options that will appeal to students? Will the price point for the plant-based options be similar, greater, or lower than the meat-based options? What is the potential impact of the switch on the food service's budget in both the short and long term?

Compatibility: Will the change require significant modifications in how the cafeteria operates, including how foods are prepared and how students experience the food options available in the cafeteria? Will the new entrées require any special kitchen equipment or food service worker skills?

Observability: How obvious will the change be to food service staff and students? Will the change be evident immediately? Will the outcome of the change, both positive and negative aspects, be highly visible to stakeholders?

Trialability: Can the change in entrée options be made incrementally over time to see how the innovation works for food service staff and students? Can adjustments and refinements be made easily? Can food service phase in more plant-based options over time, or is it important to market this change as a big, positive improvement of food service?

Relative advantage: Will this change increase student participation in the university dining services? What is the advantage with regard to student and planetary health that might be realized from the change? Will students consume healthier diets? Will the university dining service be making contributions toward reducing carbon emissions and greenhouse gases?

Simplicity: How easy will it be for the dining service administrators to explain to food service staff and students the rationale for the change? How much resistance can they expect?

APPLYING DIFFUSION OF INNOVATION CONCEPTS (*Continued*)

Example B: Changing the Physical and Social Environment to Increase Workers' Physical Activity

A worksite is looking for ways to help employees be more physically active in an effort to enhance employee health and reduce health-related costs. They are considering creating a 1.5-mile asphalt walking path around the perimeter of the worksite campus to encourage workers to be more active during the workday. Concomitant with creating this walking path is a plan to change policies and practices around break time and when the campus is open before and after work shifts. In considering this change, the company needs to consider several factors:

The cost of the change: How much will it cost to clear the land and install an asphalt path? Are there features of the current landscape (e.g., a grove of trees) that would need to be removed? Will encouraging workers to walk on campus during breaks or before and after work increase or decrease work production?

Compatibility of change: How compatible would encouraging walking on the new path be with existing company practices and policies regarding what employees do on their breaks or before and after work? How compatible would these changes be with other worksite wellness efforts?

Observability: The construction of the new walking path will be very observable; how evident will its success be at getting employees to be more active before, after, or during work? How observable will a failure be?

Trialability: Is there a possibility of a trial period before the innovation is fully implemented?

Relative advantage: How will employees and upper management view these changes? Will employees see it as too paternalistic? Will upper management see it as a positive step to keep employees healthy or will they see it as a waste of money? To what degree does the building of the pathway and the change in company policy help employees be more active, enhancing their health and reducing absenteeism?

Simplicity: How easy will it be for the company to explain the rationale for new path and change in policy to its relevant stakeholders, including workers, investors, and other community groups affected by it?

TABLE 2.2. Comparing Stages of Change and Diffusion of Innovation

Stages of change	Diffusion of innovation	Characteristic of stage
Precontemplation	—	No intention to change
Contemplation	Awareness Persuasion	Considering potential benefits/costs of change
Preparation	Decision	Preparing to take action, taking the beginning steps toward change
Action	Implementation	Change occurs
Maintenance	Confirmation	Seeking reinforcement for maintaining behavior change or innovation
Termination	Institutionalization	Change becomes the new norm

Community Change Through Community Engagement: How Change Happens in Organizations and Communities

Designing health behavior change initiatives that benefit communities is at the heart of public health (Glanz & Ammerman, 2015). For public health initiatives to be effective, they need to engage communities in the change process. *Communities* may be defined in a number of ways, including a group of people who live proximate to each other (e.g., people living in a specific area of town), functional spatial units that provide services to a group of people (e.g., people living in senior housing), groups with patterned social interaction (e.g., the congregation of a church, synagogue, or mosque), or some other symbolic unit of collective identify (e.g., veterans or LGBTQ; Minkler et al., 2008).

Methods of community change take a wide range of approaches, including those that rely on building consensus for change, such as community development, community building, and capacity building. In addition, conflict-based

INSIGHTS FOR INTERVENTIONISTS: THE UTILITY OF DOI FOR EXAMINING HOW CHANGE HAPPENS IN ORGANIZATIONS

For interventionists designing a multilevel behavior change intervention, DOI provides important insights into the factors that may facilitate or hinder innovation. It is particularly relevant to changes at the social and physical environmental levels. DOI suggests that interventionists need to (a) consider how the characteristics of an innovation may affect its acceptability by stakeholders, (b) appreciate the importance of identifying innovators or early adopters that can serve as role models for change, and (c) be aware that change in organizations and groups may progress in stages similar to how individuals work through change.

approaches, such as social action and empowerment-oriented social action, can be effective for community change (Wallerstein et al., 2015). A detailed discussion of community change is beyond the scope of this book, but a review of the key concepts and principles of community engagement as well as a description of two approaches for engaging community in creating interventions follow.

Five key concepts and principals in community engagement include community capacity, empowerment, critical consciousness, health equity, and participation (Wallerstein et al., 2015).

- **Community capacity:** The concept that a community is a unit of identity with unique characteristics that affect the community's ability to identify problems, mobilize as a community to act, and to address social and public health challenges unique to the community. The characteristics that influence community capacity include the degree to which community members actively participate in solving problems, have strong community-centric leadership and rich support networks, have a shared sense of community, history, and values, and access to power (Goodman et al., 1998).

- **Community empowerment:** A social action process that helps people gain mastery over their lives and their community by changing their social and physical environments to improve equity and quality of life. Empowerment involves approaches to positively influence individual members of the community, organizations within the community, and the community's social structure. Empowerment approaches for individuals include increasing their confidence and interest in participating in the political process. Empowerment approaches for organizations include enhancing advocacy skills and organizational effectiveness in policy change (Laverack, 2007). Community capacity stresses the importance of building on community strengths and assets, whereas empowerment stresses colearning and integrating knowledge and action.

- **Critical consciousness:** A cyclical and iterative process in which the community actively reflects on their common history and heritage. The process honors diversity and cultural humility while practicing collaborative mentorship toward positive social change.

- **Health equity:** The opportunity for all to obtain their full health potential, regardless of social position or socially determined circumstances. Working to eliminate systemic racism and identifying social determinants of health are important principles of health equity. For a community change effort to embrace this concept, resources should be allocated to community-, policy-, and system-level changes that challenge inequitable conditions affecting the health of community members.

- **Community participation:** The need to start where people are and to involve community as equals in all aspects of practice and research. Community-based participatory research (CBPR) focuses on this principal as it stresses the need for community members to create their own agenda, including identifying relevant health concerns, engaging in bidirectional learning between community members and researchers, and identifying acceptable approaches for intervention and evaluation (Wallerstein et al., 2015).

Community change is a tall order requiring dedication, commitment, time, and a sincere intent to work in partnership with community. Community change does not happen with one program or intervention or in a few years but rather requires a deep and meaningful engagement with community that is consistent over time. The commitment required for developing true community partnerships is much deeper than the commitment involved in designing behavior change interventions. Still, engagement with community is an essential aspect of any public health intervention. Two intervention-related activities, Photovoice and narrative engagement, provide examples of creative ways to engage community members in articulating and sharing their experience with health-related issues in their community.

Photovoice is an approach that engages community members in collecting data on a particular issue in their community (Catalani & Minkler, 2010). The data collected are photos taken by community members documenting how they experience and view the issue as part of their daily lives. Photovoice leaders provide cameras and skills training to help participants capture images related to the issue in question. Participants then share their photos with each other and work together to choose the images that help tell the community's story, including both the challenges that the community faces with regard to an issue and the assets the community brings to meet the challenge.

As an example, Lightfoot et al. (2019) used Photovoice to explore how immigrant Latino adolescents saw barriers to health care. They recruited 13 Latino youth from two community organizations in North Carolina. The approximate length of time living in the United States ranged from 3 to 14 years, with the majority of youth living in the country for more than 5 years. The youth were asked to generate a list of possible photo assignments related to the following topic: "What I wish my doctor knew about my life." After the group agreed on four topics, each individual youth was given a digital camera and tasked with taking photos to address the assignments. At photo discussion sessions, the youths each shared their photos and described how the images they took represented the assignment. One photo was chosen by group consensus per discussion session as a "trigger" image, best representing the assignment's task. The youth then engaged in a facilitated discussion process of the selected trigger image using the SHOWED technique (What do you See in the photo? What is really Happening in the photo? How does this relate to Our lives? Why does this situation exist? How can we become Empowered through our new understanding? What can we Do about it?; Wallerstein, 1994). The technique moved the discussion from the individual's perspective to a collective analysis of the problem with the goal of moving toward action. The final step in the Photovoice process involved holding two forums for relevant community stakeholders (one with health care providers and one with educators) where the youth shared their Photovoice findings and led stakeholders in discussions to reflect on the findings and begin to identify approaches to reduce barriers to health care and education.

The narrative engagement framework (NEF) relies on the shared experiences of the target audience to engage the larger community in designing prevention interventions (Miller-Day & Hecht, 2013). The NEF is based on the concept that for a prevention message to be effective, it must engage and connect others in a personal, relevant, and meaningful way. This approach stands in contrast to a more didactic approach that attempts to use logic and argument to convince an audience to change their behavior. The use of creating narratives, or personal stories, is key to creating narrative knowledge, a mental model, a behavioral model, and, ultimately, creating engagement in preventive health behaviors (Byrne, 2005).

Hopfer and Clippard (2011) suggested five qualities of narrative messages that make them particularly important for health interventions, including their ability to (a) overcome resistance toward the advocated health behavior, (b) engage less involved audiences, (c) reach low-knowledge audiences, (d) render complex information comprehensible, and (e) ground messages in the culture and experience of the target audience. All of these approaches are essential for creating community-level change.

The keepin' it REAL (kiR) drug prevention curriculum for adolescents is based on the NEF and is currently the most widely disseminated program of its kind in the world (Miller-Day & Hecht, 2013). kiR begins by collecting narratives, or personal stories, directly from adolescents about drugs, drug offers, drug refusals, drug use, and their perceptions of the culture of drug use in their communities.

TERMS USED IN THE NARRATIVE ENGAGEMENT FRAMEWORK

- **Narrative:** Stories organized around significant or consequential experiences, with characters undertaking some action, within a context, with implicit or explicit beginning and end points, and significance for the narrator or her or his audience

- **Narrative knowledge:** The quality of narrative messages enhancing the human capacity to construct mental models and be a significant site for individual learning

- **Mental models:** A representation of the world around us, the relationships between its various parts, and a person's intuitive perception about their own acts and the consequences of those acts in that world

- **Behavioral models:** Learning new behaviors by observation that can be incorporated into existing behavioral repertoires, change existing repertoires, or to create new behavioral repertoires

Stories are recorded and transcribed allowing cultural grounding to occur; cultural grounding is the process of identifying cultural texts and developing culture-centric messages by and for the cultural group (Hecht & Krieger, 2006). These qualitative data are then analyzed within and across narratives to identify common and patterned experiences shared by adolescents. The next step is to translate the findings into health promotion messages using the help of teen advisory teams in creating messages that have personal meaning for the adolescents and maximize their engagement. The narrative messages are then turned into student-produced videos, classroom-based discussions, and role-playing scenarios with the intent of reshaping norms, imparting narrative knowledge, and enhancing health promotive mental and behavioral models.

Both Photovoice and the NEF have at their cores the importance of hearing directly from the community to understand how they experience and respond to the issue at hand. Both engage the target audience as the primary source for data collection, allowing a connection with community that is difficult for researchers or practitioners to achieve. This approach extends the formative work conducted with stakeholders in the planning phase of interventions by actively involving community stakeholders in creating elements of the intervention. In the previous examples, Photovoice participants use their findings to inform and motivate relevant community stakeholders through forums or community meetings. In the NEF, participants produce their own curriculum, including videos or dramatization, to tell their stories.

INSIGHTS FOR INTERVENTIONISTS: THE UTILITY OF A COMMUNITY-ENGAGED APPROACH FOR EXAMINING HOW CHANGE HAPPENS IN A COMMUNITY

For interventionists wanting to use a community-engaged approach in creating interventions, keep in mind that community engagement requires time, commitment, and an appreciation for the assets and strengths that each community brings to the process. Working with and actively engaging community is essential for community-based health promotion activities. Community involvement is particularly important for positively influencing the social environment. Communities, however they are defined, are important sources for role-modeling, observational learning, establishing normative behavior, and providing social support. Involving community members in the creation of programs and interventions can help ensure that the components and strategies used are relevant and important to the community. At the same time, be realistic about what an individual intervention or community program can do. It is not realistic to believe that a single intervention or program can eliminate systemic racism or change the economic conditions of a community. But every community-based intervention has the potential and responsibility to help build community capacity, empower individuals and organizations, and work toward health equity.

Policy as a Prevention Strategy—The Multiple Streams Framework (MSF): How Change Happens in Organizations and Communities

Creating new policies and practices is another way to create change. "Policy approaches" may mean different things to different people in different contexts, however. Policy and practice change can be differentiated by "big-P Policies" and "small-p policies" (Ball, 2008). Big-P policies are formal policies adopted by an official governing body (e.g., federal, state, or local governments) or legislative action such as ordinances or executive orders. Small-p policies are those policies (often written) or practices (often not written) that communicate expected behavior of a group without any legally binding or official status. Organizations or nongovernmental agencies such as schools, worksites, or community venues often have small-p policies to communicate expectations about behaviors of the group. Even families might have unwritten practices about expected behavior.

For example, policies that change the drinking age in a specific jurisdiction, impose an industry-level tax on sugar sweetened beverages, or limit the advertising of tobacco products on television and radio represent big-P Policies. These policies typically target the macro environment, are directed at system-level change, and have the potential for significant public health impact. But such policies are often beyond the scope of behavior change interventions developed and evaluated as intervention research or community-level programming. In contrast, it is possible for an intervention research project or community programming to facilitate the development of small p policies or practices to effect change in micro environments or venues such as schools, worksites, community centers, fitness clubs, or homes. Worksites might have policies that prevent smoking on campus; schools might have a policy that restricts the types of foods that school sport teams can sell; families may have rules that prohibit watching television during mealtime. MLIs are more likely to target small-p policies rather than big-P policies because they involve interventions to be conducted and evaluated within a specific time period. However, lessons learned about communities, systems, or organizations through small-p policy change can inform and support efforts leading to big-P policy change.

Changing the policy and practice of organizations or groups is a challenging task that typically requires the buy-in and cooperation of a variety of stakeholders, a commitment to the process of building support for change, an opportune time for change, and often a single individual to act as a champion for change. The multiple streams framework (MSF) is one approach for examining these elements and the process of policy change. MSF was developed by John Kingdon in 1984 as a way to understand public policy agenda setting, but it can be helpful in thinking through how policy change happens in community-engaged behavior change interventions and programs (Kingdon, 2011).

The MSF focuses on how three categories of independent and interdependent streams interact to produce "windows of opportunity" for policy agenda-setting. The *problem stream* includes all of the potential problems (real or perceived by relevant stakeholders) that are seen as "public" or requiring some involvement from government or organizational leaders to be resolved. The problem may be objectively documented (e.g., an increase in violent crimes as documented in public safety records) or a perception of stakeholders ("It seems like there is more violence in our town"). The problems that are perceived as important may differ from stakeholder to stakeholder based on their own concerns or how they personally experience issues in the community. Public problems may reach the awareness of policy makers because of dramatic events such as community-level crises or through more personal routes such as hearing about the concerns of other community members. The important point about this stream is that multiple problems, or perceptions of problems, will exist concurrently and compete for the time and attention of potential policy makers.

The *policy stream* is made up of the ideas and potential solutions identified from experts and analysts. In this stream, myriad possibilities for policy action and inaction are identified, assessed, and narrowed down to a subset of feasible options. The important attribute of this stream is the importance for reasonable and viable public solutions for the public problems. If no reasonable policy action is available, the problem may be ignored or dismissed until a solution arises; if good policy options exist, policy-makers may feel more confident in their ability to take on the issue.

The third stream is the *political stream* or the factors that influence policy leaders' interest in and commitment to working on a problem. Factors influential in this political stream include the felt urgency by stakeholders, the strength of group advocacy campaigns or the opinions, and priorities of executives or legislators who are in power (Béland & Howlett, 2016). The political stream may ebb and flow depending on the political leaders in charge and the community groups actively engaged in forwarding their agenda.

According to Kingdon (2011), these three streams flow along different channels and remain more or less independent of one another until, at a specific point in time, a policy window (also referred to as an agenda window) opens, representing a convergence of political will that instigates a policy process. Often a policy entrepreneur (or champion for change) is required to move the policy process forward. These policy entrepreneurs are those "advocates who are willing to invest their resources-time, energy, reputation, money—to promote a position in return for anticipated future gain in the form of material, purposive, or solidary benefits" (Kingdon, 2011, p. 179).

For the intervention team considering policy change as an intervention component, these concepts from MSF (the three streams, the policy window, and the policy entrepreneur) provide insights into the potential for policy change as an effective intervention approach. For the problem stream, the intervention team may consider the following:

- What are the other problems that are likely in this community's problem stream? Is the community overloaded with problems to be solved through policy approaches? Can they pay attention to one more problem? How important is this problem relative to other problems that the community is wrestling with?

- Is it possible to link the problem that we want to solve with other problems in the stream in the hopes that a single solution might help solve multiple problems? For example, can health concerns about student e-cigarette use also be tied to concerns about student academic achievement? Can a problem related to worker health also be related to company concerns about productivity and company health care costs?

For the policy stream, the intervention team may consider the following:

- Are there good policy solutions available to address the problems? What are the most appropriate policy options to address this problem, in this community or organization, at this time? This consideration emphasizes the importance of working with an engaged community who can help determine the most appropriate strategies. It also stresses the importance of formative assessment to help understand community priorities and the ways they typically address community-level problems.

- Does the community have any prior experience successfully implementing a policy approach for a similar issue? Are there examples from other communities or organizations where a policy solution was effective in solving a problem? Communities or organizations are more likely to consider a policy solution if they have some confidence that they will be successful in achieving their goals either through their own experience or vicariously as they observe the experiences of similar organizations or communities.

For the political stream, the intervention team may consider the following:

- What is the political will for working on this problem with the policy options available at this time? Has there been some event, occurrence, or information made available that could help instigate change? Are there people in power who would get behind this problem and who agree with the potential policy options?

- Is there strong community support for this policy? Are community groups activated and ready to work for change? Is the public support for working on this problem evident to and valued by policy makers?

For the policy window or agenda window to target, the intervention team should consider the following:

- Are there obvious opportunities for pushing this agenda such as a required report, certification, or election where an elected official could garner support for their own agenda as well as a specific policy?

- Is there a time of year or organizational cycle that would provide an opportune time to push the agenda?

For an effective policy entrepreneur, the intervention team should consider the following:

- Is there a community leader or group that is well respected and positioned to champion this issue? Is there a person or a group that will be particularly important in garnering support for this issue and policy approach?

- Is this policy entrepreneur well versed on the issue and ready to invest time and resources in moving this policy forward?

Making policy can also be viewed through a diffusion of innovation lens. A policy can be seen as an innovation, and policy makers can be viewed as innovators or early adopters of change. By highlighting the characteristics that make innovations easier to adopt (e.g., how compatible changes from the new policy would be for the status quo or the relative advantage of a new approach compared with the approach being replaced) policy makers may be convinced to support the policy. Likewise, organizational and community leaders that are comfortable with risk and innovative by nature may be the policy entrepreneurs that are needed to help make policy happen.

Keep in mind that many of the health behavior theories and approaches that apply to changing individual-level behavior can be applied to policy makers. Policy makers are people too, and if interventionists can influence their opinions, motivations, and attitudes about the need for the policy, the policy maker's potential to have a positive impact on the community, or even the potential benefit to their own career by supporting the policy, the intervention team might be able to lead them to make policy or practice change. For example, local store owners might be persuaded to adopt a policy prohibiting promotions for e-cigarettes if they are convinced that the use of e-cigarettes is

INSIGHTS FOR INTERVENTIONISTS: THE UTILITY OF A POLICY APPROACH FOR EXAMINING HOW CHANGE HAPPENS IN ORGANIZATIONS, SYSTEMS, AND COMMUNITIES

Considering the following five concepts from MSF can help an intervention team decide whether using a policy or practice approach is reasonable: (a) community concern for the problem the intervention team is attempting to solve relative to other problems the community is dealing with, (b) viable policy solutions to meet the needs and match the capacity of the community, (c) the political will for solving the problem, (d) possible windows for pursuing the agenda, and (e) the availability of political and community leaders to move the agenda forward. These attributes must be considered along with the intervention group's timeline, as well as the cost and political constraints. In addition, when working directly with policy makers, keep in mind that behavior change theories may be useful in motivating policy makers' decisions.

harmful to youth in their community (susceptibility and severity), that as store owners they will not lose significant revenue as a result of the policy (benefits vs. barriers), and that the community they serve disapproves of youth using e-cigarettes (social norms and expectations).

SUMMARY

Health behavior theories are among the most important tools of a behavioral scientist and are useful for researchers and practitioners designing MLIs to promote community health. Their value in explaining health behavior has been established through research across a variety of behaviors and communities. Their importance in promoting community health has been established by showing that interventions and programs that are grounded in theory are more likely to be successful in promoting community health. This intervention design process does not recommend any specific theory; rather, it suggests that theories can be disaggregated in an effort to identify determinants that are related to the behavior of interest in the community of interest. In creating an MLI, theories that address how the process of change occurs at multiple levels may help intervention teams think through how to create intervention strategies that recognize and leverage that change process at both the individual and system level. Chapters 3 and 4 of this volume describe how both types of theories are used in designing MLIs to promote community health.

3

The Plan Phase

This chapter describes the four steps that make up the Plan Phase. This is the most important phase of the entire intervention design process because it develops the blueprint for the project, clearly documenting what health behavior the intervention will attempt to change and the mechanisms through which that change will occur. Step 1 of the Plan Phase begins by identifying a behavior-based community health problem that is relevant to the community and modifiable within the time frame of an intervention study or community program planning initiative. Identifying the determinants that are related to those behaviors in the community (Step 2 of the design process) is an essential step in designing the intervention. This chapter describes three approaches for identifying the determinants of a behavior for a specific community: using health behavior theory, examining the empirical literature, and using formative assessment in the community. It includes guidance on how to construct an evidence table to examine the empirical literature for potential determinants and a process for identifying the most relevant behavioral determinants to be the focus of the intervention. The role and importance of formative evaluation with community stakeholders to identify determinants specific to their community is covered. The chapter also describes the process of creating a conceptual model using the identified target behavior and determinants (Step 3). Step 4 ("Review the conceptual model with the evaluation team and community stakeholders") includes information on creating an intervention manual of procedures to document intervention decisions.

https://doi.org/10.1037/0000292-004
Designing Interventions to Promote Community Health: A Multilevel, Stepwise Approach,
by L. A. Lytle

An example of an intervention to reduce middle school students' consumption of sugar-sweetened beverages (SSBs) is used throughout the book to illustrate the process of designing a multilevel intervention (MLI). This hypothetical example is introduced in the Plan Phase and used to demonstrate how determinants are identified and chosen during this phase.

There are four steps to the Plan Phase:

1. Identify a behavior-based community health problem.
2. Choose the relevant behavioral determinants.
3. Create a conceptual model.
4. Review the conceptual model with the evaluation team and community stakeholders.

STEP 1: IDENTIFY A BEHAVIOR-BASED COMMUNITY HEALTH PROBLEM

What Types of Health Problems Are Well-Suited to a Multilevel, Community-Based Intervention?

The need for a community-based intervention or program can be identified in several ways. Sometimes a new problem presents itself in an urgent manner and the health community is called on to "do something"; the opioid crisis that has exploded in recent decades is an example. Handwashing and social distancing during the COVID-19 pandemic is another example of urgency. Other times, the health problems faced are long-standing and well known to the community, such as Type 2 diabetes, underage drinking, or physical inactivity. Sometimes a unique opportunity for intervention or programmatic work presents itself and becomes the impetus for change. For example, a new funding mechanism tied to a particular health problem becomes available or stakeholders who can champion the need for a particular program emerge and provide the direction and energy for creating a program. Not all health problems are well suited to community-based solutions or require MLIs, however.

The health problems that require complex MLIs are those with epidemiologic evidence that a behavior is linked to a health risk, affect multiple domains of health (including physical, mental, and social well-being), are widespread in a community, and are anticipated to persist or spread over time (Perry, 1999). The association between a behavior and a health risk needs to be confirmed by epidemiologic findings that clearly link a behavior to morbidity and mortality risk. The fact that some groups find a population behavior concerning or personally distasteful is not a reason to instigate a community-based intervention. For example, although some may find body tattoos objectionable, there is no clear evidence of health risks; therefore, it is not a health behavior that is appropriate for a community-level intervention.

Behaviors that affect multiple domains of health are good candidates for community-based health interventions because the consequences of the behavior are far-reaching. They are appropriate for MLIs because the causes and potential responses to the health behavior lie in the context of the larger social and physical environment where the behavior occurs, not just at the individual level. As an example, underage drinking is a community problem because it can affect the physical, mental, and social health of teens by increasing risk of alcohol-related injury, increasing depression, and negatively affecting social ties in the family, at school, and among peers. It is a health problem appropriate for MLIs because the etiology of underage drinking has roots in adolescents' social and physical environments where role-modeling, social reinforcement, cues, and opportunities for drinking exist (Perry, 1999). Potential solutions for addressing underage drinking include enforcing restricted sales to minors at bars and liquor stores and health education in schools to increase adolescents' awareness of the risks of drinking.

Community-based multilevel programs are also best suited for health problems that have an impact on many people in the community and are persistent problems that are likely to endure or spread. Health problems that have low prevalence rates in the community, are transient in nature, and are not likely to spread do not warrant the resources needed for a multilevel, community-based program. As an example, the low prevalence of schizophrenia in a community and the individual nature of the etiology of the disease suggest that individual, medical-based treatments are the most appropriate approaches (Perry, 1999). In comparison, depression has been estimated to affect nearly 10% of the population (Pratt & Brody, 2014), and its prevalence has increased over time. The factors suggested as potentially responsible for the population level increase in depression include systemic and community-level factors, such as lack of health insurance and economic conditions (Compton et al., 2006). Therefore, depression is an appropriate target for multilevel, community-based programs.

Often behaviors covary or occur together, and the combination of the behaviors increases disease risk. As an example, a study looking at eating, activity, and smoking behaviors in a cohort of youth followed from their sixth- to 12th-grade years found that students who reported lower activity patterns and fewer healthy food choices also reported higher levels of weekly smoking compared with students who reported higher levels of activity and healthier food choices. The results also show that the associations between the three behaviors strengthened over time, and the risk for smoking initiation increased as the youth transitioned from sixth grade to 12th grade (Lytle et al., 1995). These results suggest that there may be a health-related lifestyle risk profile. To the extent that health behaviors covary, interventions targeting general health motivations and community-, organizational-, and system-level approaches that encourage healthy behavioral patterns are appropriate. For example, a community intervention that promotes healthy food vendors or farmer's market stalls with fresh produce along a newly constructed bike path through town encourages both physical activity and healthy eating. For those designing multilevel behavior change interventions, it will be important to focus on a limited number of behaviors to design an intervention that addresses key determinants of the behaviors and to make sure that resources are not spread too thin.

What Is the Role of Community in Identifying a Health Problem?

Multilevel community health programs are done *with the community*, not just *in the community*. Health educators have long recognized the importance of starting with a community's felt need and in fostering community ownership of programs and initiatives. Community-engaged interventions have been shown to be effective in improving health behaviors and outcomes and work, in part, through their efforts to enhance community empowerment and to build community capacity (O'Mara-Eves et al., 2013). Several models for community engagement exist, including community-based participatory research, empowerment evaluation, participatory or community action research, and participatory rapid appraisal (Ahmed & Palermo, 2010). For the purpose of this book, I refer to *community engagement* as the process of working collaboratively with and through groups of people to address issues affecting the well-being of those people (Centers for Disease Control and Prevention [CDC], 1997).

Community engagement is needed throughout all the steps involved in designing multilevel behavior change interventions, including the first step of identifying a problem that is important to the community. There are times when community stakeholders, public health researchers, and practitioners all recognize a health problem and are unified in their desire to begin the process of looking for community-level solutions. Other times, the problems that the community identifies as important do not match with what public health professionals see as priority issues; likewise, health problems that may be a priority for public health professionals may not be seen as a problem within the community. This discordance needs to be addressed before effective and sustainable community solutions can be achieved.

As an example, imagine that a city health department is concerned about low measles vaccination rates for children of recent immigrants and wants to work with the community to increase rates. When speaking with the community about what the health department perceives as a problem (low vaccination rates), they learn that the immigrant group is less worried about their children getting measles and more concerned about autism. In addition, many in the community mistakenly believe that vaccinations could cause autism. The parents see measles as a minor inconvenience but experience having a child with autism as a situation affecting the entire family for life. The health department knows that ignoring the community's concerns and pressing forward with a vaccination campaign is not an option. Doing so would result in a lack of community buy-in for any type of vaccination program and would erode trust, threatening current and future initiatives. The city health department decides to proceed slowly, arranging opportunities to listen to people from the community talk about their concerns about vaccination, their fear of autism and its possible causes, and their struggles with having an autistic child. The health department

CHARACTERISTICS OF A BEHAVIOR-BASED COMMUNITY HEALTH PROBLEM

- Epidemiologic evidence confirms that the behavior causes morbidity and mortality.
- The behavior affects multiple domains of health (physical, mental, and social well-being).
- The behavior is widespread in the community.
- The behavior is anticipated to persist or spread over time.

connects families with social services as a way to offer immediate help and then begins the work of identifying members of the immigrant community to be advocates for vaccination. By working with community partners, they are able to begin educating the community on the benefits of vaccination and find solutions to reduce barriers to vaccination.

Using Charrettes to Engage Community in the Planning Process

A charrette is one approach for engaging the community in active and creative input, design, and problem-solving. A *charrette* is a collaborative planning process most often used in design and architecture that harnesses the talents and energies of all interested parties to create and support a feasible plan to bring about community development and transformation (https://www.canr.msu.edu/nci). Charrettes have their basis in community planning for neighborhood revitalization plans and were a response to the frustration, expense, and time lost when plans presented to the public were met with unhappiness or anger because community input had been lacking during the process (Lennertz et al., 2008). Charrettes have more recently been used as part of community-based participatory research as a way to help partnerships among academicians, public health professionals, and community stakeholders problem solve challenges, build partnership infrastructure, and identify strategies to move research and community health projects and programs forward (Samuel et al., 2018; Smith et al., 2020).

Charrettes can be conducted in a number of ways, but key to the process is bringing together technical experts (e.g., academic researchers or members of the intervention team from the public health or medical institutions involved) and community experts (leaders and members of the community who have the greatest experience with the health issue in their community) to deeply consider the role of their partnership and how that partnership may be used to build on the assets of the community to solve problems experienced by the community. Charrettes are typically led by a facilitator skilled in the process and involve a focused deep dive into ideas, disparate priorities, and individual visions and goals for a community health issue (Smith et al., 2020). The process works to build trust, respect, and inspiration through reflective and respectful listening and increases the chances the program will be implemented, sustained, and disseminated broadly (BaRoss, 2017).

Once the health problem has been identified and there is sufficient support from the community to develop an intervention or program, the team may begin to look for existing interventions that have been tested and found to be effective in changing the behavior of interest. A consideration of existing evidence-based interventions (EBIs) is a good place for the intervention team to start to look for interventions to adopt or adapt. Interventions that have been

EXAMPLE OF THE CHARRETTE PROCESS: THE CHAMPS PROJECT

A charrette was designed to support the work of CHAMPS, a community-based participatory research (CBPR) project with the goal of examining racial differences in treatment-related symptoms, symptom management, and treatment completion among Black and White patients with breast cancer (Samuel et al., 2018). The stakeholders involved in CHAMPS included representation from the community, academic researchers with expertise in CBPR, and medical partners. Two charrette facilitators were chosen to lead the process, one with a community perspective and one with an academic perspective.

The goal of the charrette was to move the CBPR partnership and research process forward. The process began with the stakeholders preparing a partnership overview document that included questions to encourage self-reflection and communication about a wide variety of topics, including stakeholder experience and key roles in the partnership, health disparity being addressed through the research project and its relationship to each partners' missions and goals, thoughts on recruitment and potential intervention approaches, plans for measurement, benefits to the community, and dissemination strengths. The document included a section on key questions to address in the charrette session.

The partners met for a 3-hour, in-person charrette that included (a) a facilitator-led overview to establish ground rules for a productive and safe interaction; (b) a group résumé discussion as a way to get to know each other better and increase awareness of partner skills, strengths, and organizational mission; (c) discussion of the key questions, fostering transparency, accountability, and collective problem solving of the partners; and (d) a postcharrette evaluation form. The end product of the charrette was a summary report prepared by the cofacilitators; the CHAMPS partnership reviewed the report and the recommendations that emerged from the in-person charrette session. The charrette process increased transparency, accountability, and trust among partners; identified potential challenges and solutions to project objectives; and functioned as a catalyst for continued dialogue and capacity-building among the CHAMPS partnership (Samuel et al., 2018).

tested in similar communities, use approaches that appear potentially feasible in the new community, and have shown some level of effectiveness may be good candidates. An important criterion for deciding to adopt or adapt an existing EBI is the similarity in the determinants targeted in the EBI and the determinants that are related to the behavior in the new community. Therefore, the next step in the intervention design process, "Choose the relevant behavioral determinants," is an important step even if the team decides to use or adapt an existing EBI rather than design a new intervention or program. Chapter 7 provides an overview and guidance for adapting EBIs.

STEP 2: CHOOSE THE RELEVANT BEHAVIORAL DETERMINANTS

What Are Determinants, and Why Are They Important?

Before work on creating the intervention begins, the team needs a good understanding of what factors are related to, or predictive of, the behavior. These factors are called *determinants*. The identification of determinants is crucial to the design of health behavior interventions because the objective of the intervention will be to change the determinants that serve to support and reinforce the targeted behavior. The overall goal of the intervention can be either to increase a healthy behavior or decrease a risky behavior. Determinants can help predict healthy behaviors (e.g., what factors are related to higher levels of physical activity in older individuals?) and risky health behaviors (e.g., what factors are related to the initiation of vaping in young adults?).

It is also important to focus on determinants of behaviors rather than directly focusing on a health outcome because community-based interventions will attempt to change behavior and the systems and organizations that influence behavior. Although the ultimate goal of a health behavior intervention is the improvement in some biological or physiological outcome to reduce morbidity and mortality, behavior change is the most proximal predictor of a health outcome in multilevel community interventions. As an example, a community intervention may have as its ultimate goal to reduce the proportion of community members with elevated HbA1c (a biomarker for elevated risk for Type 2 diabetes). However, because the study team is testing a community-based rather than a pharmacological or medical intervention approach, they will first need to identify the behaviors that are associated with risk for Type 2 diabetes in their population of interest (likely dietary and activity-related behaviors) and the factors or determinants influencing those behaviors. They design their intervention to positively influence those determinants and behavioral outcomes and will evaluate the success of their intervention based on those outcomes. Change in the proportion of the population with elevated HbA1c may also be assessed if time and resources permit. However, often community-based MLIs are not adequately resourced, large enough, or long enough to evaluate changes in morbidity or mortality. Yet, with adequate epidemiologic evidence to causally link the behavior to disease risk, behavior change is recognized as an important outcome.

CHOOSING MORE THAN ONE BEHAVIORAL OUTCOME

There are times when a study or project targets change on two behavioral outcomes within the same intervention. For example, a team may want to see whether their school-based intervention to reduce the consumption of sugar-sweetened beverages is effective in reducing intake in both children and adults in the school. Or they may want to see if their worksite wellness intervention is effective in promoting walking during break time and increasing consumption of fruits and vegetables. The CATCH study, described in Chapter 1 of this volume, is an example of a study that focused on eating, activity, and preventing the initiation of smoking in youth in a single intervention but with multiple intervention components and determinants targeting each behavior.

Although it may be possible to have two or more primary behavioral outcomes, keep in mind that the determinants of the behavior may be different for different population groups (children vs. adults) and for different behaviors (walking during break time at work vs. fruit and vegetable consumption), and behavior-specific determinants may require unique intervention approaches. Targeting more than one behavior in a single intervention requires a consideration of the time and resources available. Often teams will choose a single behavior as their primary outcome and designate other behaviors as secondary outcomes as a way to prioritize resources.

Possible determinants of a behavior are identified through three approaches: (a) using behavioral theory, (b) examining the empirical research, and (c) learning from and listening to the community. The next section details how each of these approaches is used to identify possible determinants.

Using Theory to Identify Potential Determinants

Behavioral theories are a good place to start to identify potential determinants to be targeted in a community-based intervention. Theories or models of behavior change are made up of a set of interrelated concepts or constructs organized with the intent of explaining or predicting some outcome (Glanz et al., 2015b). For the purpose of designing interventions, constructs from theories represent potential determinants of behavior. Theory can help identify the determinants in people's individual, social, and physical environments that may be facilitating or hindering their ability to make healthy choices. Chapter 2 presents an overview of theory and describes three commonly used theories to explain or predict behavior.

A basic understanding of behavior change theories provides the intervention team with some sense of the determinants that have been shown to predict or explain health behavior. Theory is particularly helpful when the empirical research on a specific behavior or population group is lacking; one of the strengths of a theory is its generalizability. In addition, knowledge of theoretical constructs may be helpful in naming or categorizing information obtained through the review of the empirical research and formative evaluation. Theoretical constructs become part of the lexicon used to describe to others the mechanism by which the intervention attempts to change behavior and helps in replication and dissemination of interventions.

The job of the interventionist is to identify potentially helpful behavioral theories and unpack those theories to identify constructs or determinants that might help predict behavior in the population that they are working with. The ability to deconstruct theories into constructs is especially important with MLIs because theories may include constructs that are influential across one or more environments. Table 3.1 lists constructs organized by the individual, social, or physical environment from the theories described in Chapter 2 (specifically, the health belief model, theory of planned behavior, and social cognitive theory) that may be useful as intervention determinants. In designing MLIs, it is important to identify determinants across multiple environments. Choosing from just the individual environment or just the physical environment is unlikely to be a successful strategy.

Community-based MLIs are not designed to test theory; rather, they draw on theory as a tool for designing interventions to be implemented and evaluated in real-world settings. As the intervention or program planning team reviews potential theories, keep in mind that the overall purpose of this activity in the Plan Phase is to identify determinants that might be important to include in the intervention design. It is not important to become experts on theory or theory measurement. It easy to get lost in the nuance and detail of behavior change theories. The nomenclature can get confusing because different theories may use different terms to describe the same constructs. As an example, *perceived*

TABLE 3.1. Theoretical Constructs Organized by Environment

Individual environment	Social environment	Physical environment
Perceived susceptibility (HBM)	Cues to action (HBM)	Cues to action (HBM)
Perceived severity (HBM)	Subjective norm (TPB)	Barriers in the physical environment (SCT, HBM, TPB)
Perceived benefits (HBM, SCT)	Normative beliefs (SCT)	
Perceived barriers (HBM, SCT)	Observational learning (SCT)	Opportunities in the physical environment (SCT, HBM, TPB)
Self-efficacy (HBM, SCT)		
Perceived control (TPB)	Social support (SCT, HBM, TPB)	Reinforcements or disincentives in the physical environment (SCT)
Perceived social support (SCT)	Reinforcements or disincentives in the social environment (SCT)	
Intention (TPB, SCT)		
Knowledge (SCT)		
Outcome expectations (SCT)		
Behavioral skills (SCT)		

Note. HBM = health belief model (Becker, 1974); SCT = social cognitive theory (Bandura, 1986); TPB = theory of planned behavior (Ajzen, 1991).

barriers can be similar to *lack of self-efficacy* or *lack of perceived control*. Don't let this confusion become a roadblock; the ability to assign labels to determinants will become clearer with a review of the empirical literature and formative assessment. In addition, there are many sources of information on measuring theoretical constructs as part of program evaluation and intervention research that will help the team name determinants. Chapter 6 of this volume on the Evaluate Phase provides some background on measuring determinants across multiple environments.

It is important to note that health behavior theories generally see individual and population characteristics such as age, gender, ethnicity, socioeconomic status, and income levels as factors that describe the sample or may moderate the relationships among determinants, health behavior, and health outcomes. These factors are typically included as variables in analytic models testing the relationship but are not included as constructs causally related to behavior change. There are occasions when an intervention will try to positively and directly affect the income levels of the target audience (e.g., microfinancing interventions to help women in developing countries start businesses; Leatherman et al., 2012).

Using the Empirical Research to Identify Possible Determinants of the Behavior

An important step in understanding the determinants of behavior is to identify published articles documenting links between the health-related behavior of interest and factors associated with or predictive of the behavior. The literature review should prioritize intervention studies but will likely include longitudinal and cross-sectional studies. The review can be limited by using search terms that focus on the specific behavior of interest as well as the population of interest (e.g., *screen time, adolescents*) or may include behaviors that are more broadly related to a specific behavioral topic (e.g., *sedentary behavior, screen time, physical inactivity, television time, adolescents*). If there is a great deal of research on a topic, more specificity will help to reduce the number of articles that show up in the literature review. If there is little published on the topic, then a broader search might need to be conducted, including related behaviors and a larger population segment. For example, a behavior that is newly recognized as a health problem, such as vaping or e-cigarette use, may require looking across a wide population segment (both adults and adolescents) and may need to draw inference from studies on cigarette smoking because published research on the vaping and e-cigarettes is just beginning to emerge. Review articles may be helpful in identifying articles to include, but it is best to review the original articles to identify details on the determinants of the behavior. Because the literature on most health behaviors is multidisciplinary, a search of the public health, medical, sociological, psychological, and other disciplines will likely be needed; searching PubMed (https://pubmed.ncbi.nlm.nih.gov/) or APA PsycInfo (https://psycnet.apa.org/) will typically bring up sources across these disciplines. A reference librarian will also be helpful in this search process.

Timelines and other resources will put some limits on examining the empirical research. At some point, the team will need to decide that they have an adequate set of articles to examine in more detail. The set of articles to review in detail can be chosen by (a) identifying the articles that most closely match the health behavior in which the team is specifically interested (e.g., screen time vs. sedentary behavior; weight loss vs. weight maintenance), (b) identifying articles that include a study sample that is closely related to the population of interest (e.g., adolescents between that ages of 10 and 18 vs. youth aged 5–18; weight maintenance in young adults vs. all adults), (c) identifying articles that have been published in the past 10 years (more recent publications likely reflect the current science and improved measurement approaches), (d) prioritizing quantitative over qualitative work (the team will be conducting their own qualitative work with their specific population), and (e) prioritizing intervention research and longitudinal studies over cross-sectional work (a more rigorous study design increases one's confidence in the causal association between a determinant and a health outcome). Be aware that a great deal of the work on health behavior is cross-sectional and may be important to include despite study design limitations.

For some practice-based groups, conducting a thorough literature review may seem overwhelming. Be realistic about what the team can accomplish. Review articles may be the best place to start to identify relevant articles. In addition, look for position papers, white papers, or overviews of the behavior of interest. For example, the CDC publishes State Action Guides such as the

OVERVIEW OF SIMPLE STUDY DESIGNS

Intervention study design: A study designed to evaluate the effectiveness of an intervention. At a minimum, baseline measures of key variables must be collected before the intervention activities begin and after intervention activities end. Additional measurement periods allow an examination of the trajectory of change overtime. Well-designed intervention studies that include a control group can establish causality or confirm within reasonable doubt that the change in outcome was the result of the intervention.

Longitudinal study design: A study that includes multiple measurement periods assessing the same set of variables without an attempt to intervene on any outcome. A longitudinal study design will allow an examination of the trajectory of change in variables over time and may establish a temporal order.

Cross-sectional study design: A study that measures both determinants and outcomes at only one point in time. Correlations or associations between variables can be evaluated in a cross-sectional study, but it is impossible to establish a causal relationship.

2018 State Action Guides on Fruits and Vegetables (CDC, 2018), which includes information on the health benefits of eating fruits and vegetables as well as factors associated with consumption.

In addition, look for professional organizations or federal agencies that may have written guidelines providing a summary of the behavior and related risk factors. For example, in the United States, the Department of Health and Human Services and the U.S. Department of Agriculture publish the U.S. Dietary Guidelines every 5 years, which includes a great deal of documentation on eating behaviors (U.S. Department of Agriculture, 2020). Similarly, the Office of Disease Prevention and Health Promotion publishes the Physical Activity Guidelines for Americans with details surrounding activity-related behaviors (U.S. Department of Health and Human Services, 2018) and the Surgeon General publishes regular reports on smoking and tobacco use (CDC, n.d.-d). Using such existing documents can be a good place to begin to identify possible behavioral determinants that may be relevant for the community and population.

Creating an Evidence Table

The articles that the intervention team has identified will be used to develop an evidence table. The purpose of an evidence table is to outline the evidence for the impact of determinants on the behavior of interest so that team members can make informed decisions about which determinants to target in the intervention. Table 3.2 shows the evidence table shell.

The title of the evidence table describes the behavior that the team is planning to address through its intervention work and the target population. Each row of the evidence table represents one determinant; therefore, there may be multiple rows from a single research article if multiple determinants are included in the research. The rows are organized by the three environments that were previously described as making up the multilevel framework: (a) individual environment, (b) social environment, and (c) physical environment.

Teams will examine each article included in the literature review and identify the determinants that were evaluated. Sometimes the authors of the research might identify a theoretical basis for their etiological or intervention work and use related constructs to label determinants. For example, the authors might use the term *self-efficacy* to represent attitudes about confidence to perform a behavior; self-efficacy is used as the label for the determinant on the evidence table. Other times, some translation of the study's findings into a construct or a determinant needs to occur for its inclusion in the evidence table. For example, qualitative research with individuals participating in focus groups might reveal that the participants would like to eat a healthier diet but do not know how to do menu planning and that their cooking skills are limited. For inclusion on the evidence table, this sentiment needs to be translated into a determinant, likely *behavioral skills*.

TABLE 3.2. Evidence Table: Shell

Behavior: _____ ; Target Population: _____

Determinant	Specific behavior	Type of evidence	Population	Sample size	Findings	Reference	Notes	Scoring
				Individual-level environment				Specific behavior = Evidence = Population = Sample size = Findings = Changeability = Total score =
				Social-level environment				Specific behavior = Evidence = Population = Sample size = Findings = Changeability = Total score =
				Physical-level environment				Specific behavior = Evidence = Population = Sample size = Findings = Changeability = Total score =

Starting with the individual-level environment, fill in the evidence table for each determinant including the following:

1. **Determinant:** What determinant or factor was examined in the article for its association with the health behavior of interest? The article may use some other term to identify this determinant, such as *independent variable, exposure, construct, risk factor,* or *factor.*

2. **Specific behavior:** What specific behavioral outcome was assessed? It may be helpful to include how the behavior was measured.

3. **Type of evidence:** Was the association between the determinant and the behavior assessed cross-sectionally, longitudinally, or through an intervention study? Cross-sectional evidence provides the weakest evidence.

4. **Population:** What was the population group included in the study? Include information on the age of the population, geographic location of the study, and other relevant characteristics of the group.

5. **Sample size:** How many individuals were included in the study? If the study included a group-level intervention (for example schools, worksites, churches) how many groups were included? How many people were included in the final analysis? Was there significant attrition if a longitudinal or intervention study was used?

6. **Findings:** What were the study's findings regarding the association between the determinant and the behavior? How strong were the associations, and were they consistent across the timepoints evaluated? Are findings presented for subgroups? If so, what were the findings?

7. **Reference:** What is the citation for this article?

8. **Notes:** What else would the team like to remember about this determinant or study?

9. **Scoring:** Scoring provides a way to help decide which determinants should be targeted in the intervention and is described later.

The team continues to fill out the table, moving to determinants from the social and physical environments.

Once all of the determinants have been entered into the evidence table, the next step is to score each determinant on six aspects using the questions shown in Table 3.3. The scoring activity is not meant to be a rigorous analysis of the "best" determinants but rather to facilitate team decision making regarding the most relevant determinants to choose. Higher points are given for determinants that are (a) evaluated with a behavior that most closely fits the behavior to be targeted in the current study, (b) evaluated in an intervention study, (c) evaluated with a population that is most like the population to be targeted in the current study, (d) evaluated with a large sample size, (e) found to have strong statistical significance with the behavior being studied, and (f) estimated to be

TABLE 3.3. Six Elements for Scoring Determinants From an Evidence Table

Element	Question	Score
Specific behavior	How close was the behavior studied in this article to the behavior that you intend to study?	0. Related behavioral area but not the same behavior 1. Similar behavior 2. Exact behavior
Type of evidence	Was the association between the determinant and the behavior assessed cross-sectionally, longitudinally, or through an intervention study?	0. Cross-sectional study 1. Longitudinal study without an intervention 2. Intervention study
Population	How similar is the population studied in the article and the population in your study?	0. Very different population 1. Similar population 2. Very similar population
Sample size	How many people or groups were included in the study?	0. Small sample size (pilot or qualitative work) 1. Medium sample size 2. Large sample size
Findings	What were the study's findings regarding the association between the determinant and the behavior? Are findings presented for subgroups? If so, what were the findings?	0. No statistically significant relationship found between the determinant and the behavior for any assessment period 1. Some statistically significant associations found, but weak or inconsistent across assessment periods 2. Strong statistical significance demonstrated
Changeability	How likely is it that an intervention can be developed that could change this determinant with the time and resources available to the team?	0. Not very likely 1. Probable 2. Very likely
Total Score		Add up the points. Possible range: 0–12

a determinant that would be possible to change given the time and resources available to the team. Scores for each determinant will range from 0 to 12.

Example Evidence Table: Healthy Teens, Healthy Planet

As already noted, throughout this book, I use an example of a hypothetical school-based program to decrease consumption of SSBs in middle school students (Grades 5–8, ages 11–15) as a way to illustrate the design process. Exhibit 3.1 provides background on the rationale and impetus for the program to be developed. Also, although this program is referred to as "Healthy Teens,

EXHIBIT 3.1

Rationale and Impetus for the Healthy Teens, Healthy Planet School-Based Intervention

Leaders of the Chronic Disease Prevention Branch of a state health department and public health researchers from an academic institution in the state are concerned about the increasing prevalence of obesity in school-age children. School leaders in the state have also expressed a concern about rising obesity rates in students, particularly middle school adolescents.

A state health department representative and a public health researcher meet with the school superintendent and other school representatives to assess their interest in participating in a pilot intervention to help reduce obesity in middle school students. The school district approached serves 37,000 students, 70% of whom qualify for free or reduced lunch, has 14 schools with students in Grades 6 through 8, and is located within a major metropolitan area. Investigators from the health department and the academic institution propose to apply for a R34 Planning Grant Program from the National Institutes of Health to fund pilot intervention work with the involvement of the school district. If the pilot program is successful, a more rigorous evaluation will be planned.

Before the school district agrees to participate, it recommends that the investigators have conversations with school staff, including teachers, school nurses, school food service staff, teachers from the physical education department, and parent groups to assess their level of interest in obesity as a health risk for students, obtain their insights on factors that may be related to the increasing incidence of obesity in their school district, and to hear their ideas on appropriate intervention approaches. From these conversations, an intervention team made up of members from the health department, academic researchers, principals, a food service director, teachers, and parents emerges. The team agrees that the focus of the intervention will be to reduce student consumption of SSBs at school. One middle school, with students in Grades 6 through 8, is chosen as the pilot school.

Healthy Planet" in this chapter for clarity, this name would not be formally established by the intervention team until the team members finalize the specific objectives to focus on and intervention strategies to use. This would occur as part of Step 6 in the Create Phase (Chapter 4). This section illustrates how an evidence table for this project is created and scored. Note that this is just an example of creating an evidence table to illustrate the process. A literature review on the topic of SSB consumption in adolescents would result in many more articles.

The academic members of the intervention team are tasked with doing a literature search looking for published research from the past 15 years that examine the factors related to adolescent intake of SSB. Although they know that their intervention will be school based, they consider having a family component. Therefore, they decide to include research that focuses on school and families. They decide to exclude qualitative research because most qualitative research uses small sample sizes providing limited generalizability of the findings and because quantitative studies using comparable populations are available. In addition, the team will be conducting its own formative work, including qualitative research with their target population. After doing a literature search and reviewing the abstracts, the team identifies six published articles to include in the evidence table:

1. A study by Blum et al. (2008) reported the results of a school-based intervention in Maine, which hypothesized that changing the types of beverages available in vending machines and on a la carte lines would positively influence students' consumption of SSBs.

2. A study by Ezendam et al. (2010) with Dutch adolescents aged 12 to 13 examined the longitudinal relationships between family rules about SSB consumption and adolescents' perceptions about their ability to reduce their SSB consumption at baseline and change in daily SSB consumption between baseline and 4 months.

3. A cross-sectional study by Johnson et al. (2009) in middle schools in the United States examined the relationship between the number of vending machine slots selling SSBs, venues in the school where SSBs were available and student consumption of SSB.

4. A cross-sectional study by Bauer et al. (2011) examined the relationship between parental intake of SSB and the availability of SSB in the home and adolescent girls' average monthly intake of SSB. This study occurred with girls aged 14 to 20 from Minnesota and one of their parents.

5. A cross-sectional study by Lally et al. (2011) conducted with adolescents aged 16 to 19 from the United Kingdom examined the relationship between attitudes about consuming SSBs and their beliefs about consumption patterns of their peers and the average number of SSBs they consumed in a week.

6. A clustered randomized intervention trial by Gray et al. (2016) in which schools randomized to the intervention condition received a classroom-based nutrition education curriculum focusing on reducing perceived barriers to making healthy beverage choices at school. Schools randomized to the control condition received the standard science curriculum. School-level differences in average daily student-level intake of SSBs was assessed as the outcome. The sample included 10 middle schools and 1,136 students from the New York City area.

Table 3.4 shows a sample evidence table produced from the review of these studies. In some cases, the determinants were "labeled" and specifically evaluated in their respective studies; other times, the determinants need to be labeled by the intervention team working on the evidence table. As an example, Ezendam et al. (2010) asked students about their perceptions of how difficult it would be to drink fewer SSBs and the likelihood that they would be successful in drinking fewer SSBs. They created a variable measuring those perceptions and labeled the variable *perceived behavioral control* (PBC), a construct from the theory of

TABLE 3.4. Sample Evidence Table for the Healthy Teens/Healthy Planet Intervention to Reduce the Intake of Sugar-Sweetened Beverages (SSBs)

Behavior: Consumption of SSBs.　　**Population/setting:** Adolescents aged 12 to 18 in a large urban school district.

Determinant	Specific behavior	Type of evidence	Population	Sample size	Findings	Reference	Notes	Scoring
				Individual-level environment				
PBC (difficulty of drinking fewer SSBs; likelihood of success in drinking less)	Change in average daily SSB consumption—food frequency	Longitudinal study (baseline and 4-month follow-up measures)	Dutch adolescent students, aged 12–13 years	$N = 348$ adolescents	High (vs. low) PBC to reduce SSB consumption at Time 1 was related to decreased consumption at time 2, AOR = 0.53 [CI: 0.30, 0.97]	Ezendam et al. (2010)		Specific behavior = 2 Evidence = 1 Population = 1 Sample size = 1 Findings = 1 Changeability = 1 Total score = 7
Attitudes (SSB good/bad for health; sensible/ foolish choice)	Average number of SSBs consumed in a week (survey)	Cross-sectional study	Students from the United Kingdom, aged 16–19 years	$N = 264$ students	Attitudes were not significantly related to SSBs; standardized betas ranged from 0.05 ($p = .46$) to 0.10 ($p = .19$)	Lally et al. (2011)		Specific behavior = 2 Evidence = 0 Population = 1 Sample size = 1 Findings = 0 Changeability = 1 Total score = 5
Perceived barriers (difficulty resisting SSB, pricing, making healthy choices)	Average daily intake of SSBs (survey)	Cluster-randomized intervention trial	Students from New York City public schools, Grades 6–7; 90% of the students were Black or Hispanic	Ten middle schools (five intervention, five control): $N = 1,136$ students	Perceived barriers mediated the relationship between the intervention and SSB consumption ($p < .05$).	Gray et al. (2016)	Secondary data analysis	Specific behavior = 2 Evidence = 2 Population = 2 Sample size = 2 Findings = 2 Changeability = 2 Total score = 12

Social-level environment

Construct	Measure	Study design	Population	N	Findings	Citation	Scoring
Observational learning (parental intake of regular soft drinks)	Adolescent average monthly intake of "regular soda pop", assessed with question on student survey	Cross-sectional study	Girls from Minnesota, aged 14–20 and one parent; 71% non-White population	$N = 253$ parent-child dyads	Parental soft drink intake was positively related to girls' intake of soda pop in multivariate adjusted analysis ($B = 0.30, p = .005$)	Bauer et al. (2011)	Specific behavior = 1 Evidence = 0 Population = 1 Sample size = 1 Findings = 2 Changeability = 0 Total score = 5
Descriptive norm (perceptions of peers' SSB consumption)	Average number of SSBs consumed in a week (survey)	Cross-sectional study	Students from the United Kingdom, aged 16–19 years	$N = 264$ students	Descriptive norms were positively related to SSB consumption ($B = 0.41, p < .01$)	Lally et al. (2011)	Specific behavior = 2 Evidence = 0 Population = 1 Sample size = 1 Findings = 2 Changeability = 2 Total score = 8
Family food rules (allowed to drink as much SSB as desired at home)	Change in average daily SSB consumption (food frequency)	Longitudinal study (baseline and 4-month follow-up measures)	Dutch adolescent students, aged 12–13 years	$N = 348$ adolescents	Perceived restriction of consumption (restricted vs. not restricted was related to decreased consumption at Time 2, $AOR = 0.54$ [CI: 0.32, 0.91]	Ezendam et al. (2010)	Specific behavior = 2 Evidence = 1 Population = 1 Sample size = 1 Findings = 1 Changeability = 0 Total score = 6

(continues)

TABLE 3.4. Sample Evidence Table for the Healthy Teens/Healthy Planet Intervention to Reduce the Intake of Sugar-Sweetened Beverages (SSBs) (Continued)

Determinant	Specific behavior	Type of evidence	Population	Sample size	Findings	Reference	Notes	Scoring
Physical-level environment								
Availability of SSB in the home (one question on the availability of soft drinks in the home from a parent survey)	Adolescents' average monthly intake of "regular soda pop"; assessed with question on student survey	Cross-sectional study	Girls from Minnesota, aged 14–20 and one parent. 71% non-White population	$N = 253$ parent–child dyads	The availability of SSBs in the home was positively associated with girls' monthly intake of SSBs ($B = 0.31$, $p = .003$ in multivariate adjusted analysis)	Bauer et al. (2011)		Specific behavior = 1 Evidence = 0 Population = 1 Sample size = 1 Findings = 2 Changeability = 0 Total score = 5
Availability of SSB in school (no. of vending machine slots and SSB venues at school)	SSB consumption at school (student survey)	Cross-sectional study	Middle school students in the United States	$N = 9,151$ students in 64 schools	Schools with higher "exposure" (availability) of SSBs had a higher proportion of students reporting any SSB consumption ($B = -.157$, $p < .001$)	Johnson et al. (2009)	School = unit of analysis School policy was predictive of SSB exposure.	Specific behavior = 1 Evidence = 0 Population = 2 Sample size = 2 Findings = 2 Changeability = 2 Total score = 9
Availability of SSBs in school (types of beverages in vending and a la carte program)	Average daily SSB consumption (food frequency, pre–post intervention)	Intervention study, school-level nonrandom assignment	Public high schools in Maine	Three control schools: $n = 221$ students; four intervention schools: $n = 235$ students	No significant differences between intervention and control groups in change in SSB consumption from baseline to follow-up	Blum et al. (2008)	Very small, selective sample	Specific behavior = 2 Evidence = 2 Population = 1 Sample size = 1 Findings = 0 Changeability = 2 Total score = 8

Note. AOR = adjusted odds ratio; CI = confidence interval; PBC = perceived behavioral control.

planned behavior. The results that they present report on the association they found between PBC and change in daily consumption of SSB. Students reporting higher PBC at Time 1 reported a greater decrease in SSB consumption at Time 2 compared with students reporting lower PBC at Time 1. On the other hand, Bauer et al. (2011) examined the relationships between parental soft drink intake and their daughters' intake of "regular soda pop" but did not attach a label to "parental soft drink intake." On the basis of social cognitive theory, the creators of the evidence table translate this variable into a determinant representing *observational learning*. Attaching meaningful labels to broad concepts is important because eventually these determinants will be translated into variables and evaluated as correlates or predictors of behavior in analytic models.

The evidence table is set up to guide the development of an MLI. Three determinants were identified for each of the three environmental levels, and several studies provided information on determinants from more than one level. For example, Bauer et al. (2011) reported on the relationship between parental role-modeling (from the social environment) and SSBs as well as on the relationship between the availability of SSBs in the home (from the physical environment) and SSB consumption. In addition, inclusion in the evidence table of how the determinant and the behaviors were assessed provides detail that is helpful in understanding the context of the relationship between the determinant and behavior. As an example, in the study by Johnson et al. (2009), information in the evidence table for the determinant *availability of SSB in schools* includes that availability was assessed by counting the number of vending machine slots in the schools and the number of venues in the school where SSBs were available. Behavior was assessed via a student survey asking about beverage and snack consumption during the school day (Johnson et al., 2009).

Table 3.4 also shows the hypothetical scoring of each determinant considering the specificity of behavior to the intervention team's behavioral target, the type of evidence, population, sample size, findings, and their estimation of the ability to change the determinant in their population. As an example, the determinant that scored the highest was from the study by Gray et al. (2016). The behavioral outcome they studied (i.e., average daily intake of SSBs) is the same outcome that this study is proposing to use to evaluate the effectiveness of the intervention. In addition, the study was an intervention study that examined how change in "perceived barriers" (operationalized as difficulty resisting SSB, pricing, and making healthy choices) was related to change in the outcome. The population studied by Gray et al. matched the population to be studied (students in middle school) and included a large sample size (10 schools and more than 1,000 students). Their findings showed that change in perceived barriers was a statistically significant mediator of the intervention and student intake of SSBs. Finally, the team members scored *changeability* as a 2 because they believed it was possible for their team to create an intervention that could be successful in reducing students' perceptions of barriers. The determinant *attitudes* from the Lally et al. article (2011) received one of the lowest scores due to the cross-sectional nature of the study (limiting the strength of the evidence produced), a population that was slightly older and from another culture, a small sample size, and study results that showed no association between attitudes as measured and the behavioral outcome. This low score suggests that this determinant is not a strong enough candidate to be included in the intervention planning work. Notice that the determinant *descriptive norm* from the same study (Lally et al., 2011) received a higher score because statistically significant findings between descriptive norms and behavior were found, and the study teams felt that changing descriptive norms would be possible through their intervention.

On the basis of this hypothetical exercise, four determinants emerge with the highest scores: PBC (individual environment), perceived barriers (individual environment), descriptive norms (social environment), and availability of beverages at school (physical environment). The determinants that emerged through the scoring are well represented in behavior change theories, and the team members used their knowledge of theory and scoring as a way to inform their decisions. Knowing that adolescents are less motivated by health risks points away from choosing determinants from the health belief model, whereas recognition of the importance of adolescents' social environment points toward constructs from the theory of planned behavior and social cognitive theory. Because the intervention is school based, attention to reducing barriers and creating opportunities in the physical environment aligns with both social cognitive theory and issues of perceived control from theory of planned behavior. This evidence table and the scoring of the determinants will be set aside until the formative evaluation is conducted.

Using Formative Evaluation to Identify Possible Behavioral Determinants

Once the team has a good grasp of potential theoretical constructs that might be useful and the evidence table is complete, the final source to consider in identifying potential determinants is the community with which the team will be working. It is unlikely that the specific community will be represented in the empirical literature unless the team has been working with the same community on the same behavioral issues and the findings have been published in the empirical literature. If that is the case, this step of identifying determinants should be quick and easy for the team. For most teams, however, formative assessment with community stakeholders will be necessary to understand how the community experiences and perceives the health problem, related health behavior, and behavioral determinants. Formative assessment with the community differs from but complements the charrette work done earlier in the community because this formative work drills deeper into specifics of how the community experiences a behavior, whereas charrettes are important for the broader intention of engaging a community.

Formative evaluation includes any data collection done to help "form" an intervention. Formative evaluation can and does occur during all phases of the intervention design process, from identifying determinants to evaluating the outcome. During the Plan Phase, formative evaluation is specifically conducted to help determine the focus of the intervention and answer the following questions: What determinants may drive behavior in this community? How does this community experience and think about this behavior and the factors that influence it? Formative assessment done after the intervention has been completed helps the team learn from the experience to help form the next iteration of the intervention, answering the following questions: How does the intervention need to be revised? What went well, and not so well, in this version of the intervention? Did the intervention work better for some subgroups than other subgroups? Often process data collected during the intervention are a source of formative evaluation. Process evaluation involves collecting data on how the intervention is delivered and is covered in more depth in the Implement Phase (Chapter 5, this volume).

Conducting a formative evaluation ensures that the team developing the intervention is connected with and understands the experiences and needs of the target community group. Building on the charrette process, formative assessment helps the intervention team learn more about the community, including its assets, challenges, history, and structure. Alliances are built, and community members who will be part of the intervention and evaluation teams are identified. Formative evaluation greatly increases the potential for successful implementation and dissemination of the intervention or program because the intervention is built in the community with engaged community partners rather than dropped into place from an outside group. Formative evaluation is also helpful in learning the language and terms that the target audience uses to talk about the health issue and behavior. That knowledge can help tailor the intervention materials and communication tools to be developed.

Formative evaluation may be quantitative (using close-ended questions in surveys) or qualitative (using open-ended questions in interviews or focus groups); collecting both types of data is ideal. Occasionally, existing survey data are available to provide some information on the health issue, behavior, and determinants of the behavior in the population of interest. These data are more likely to be available in groups that have previously been studied, communities near universities, and communities near larger urban areas. As an example, the Minnesota Department of Education has administered and reported on the Minnesota Student Survey for the past 30 years (Minnesota Department of Health, n.d.). Students respond to questions on school climate, bullying, out-of-school activities, health and nutrition, emotional and mental health, relationships, substance use, and more. Data obtained are available at the state, county, and district level. Sometimes regional data that includes information on the target population can be obtained from national data sources. As an example, the CDC's Behavioral Risk Factor Surveillance System (CDC, n.d.-a) collects behavioral health risk data for adults at the state and local levels.

The behaviors assessed include tobacco use, alcohol consumption, sleep, immunization, oral health, and many others. Likewise, the Youth Risk Behavior Surveillance System administered by the CDC (n.d.-e) includes quantitative data from representative samples of ninth- through 12th-grade students on a variety of behaviors, including unintentional injuries and violence, sexual behaviors, alcohol and other drug use, tobacco use, unhealthy dietary behaviors, and inadequate physical activity. The data can be accessed at the levels of national, state, and large urban districts. Community health assessments might be useful and available in many places across the country, either through public health infrastructure or nonprofit hospitals via the Community Health Needs Assessments required by the Affordable Care Act (CDC, n.d.-b). The advantages of using existing survey sources include the savings in time and money and the increased likelihood that the measurement tools used in the surveys have demonstrated reliability and validity.

However, existing surveys may not be specific enough to the target population group or to the needs of the project. In those cases, new survey data may be needed. The advantage of creating a new survey is that the questions asked, and the population surveyed, can be highly specific to the needs of the project. However, writing survey questions, obtaining consent, collecting data according to a protocol, and having the time and expertise for data analysis are significant challenges, especially for busy health practitioners. Creating survey items is challenging, and information on how to develop and test them is beyond the scope of this book; Fowler (2014) and Saris and Gallhofer (2014) are excellent resources on this topic. Sometimes very short, targeted surveys can be developed to be administered in conjunction with focus groups or interviews or for a very specific group of stakeholders. However, the sample sizes used for formative assessment are often small, making confidentiality especially important.

Key informant interviews and focus groups are two qualitative approaches for formative evaluation. These methods allow the project team to ask specific questions of the most relevant stakeholders. Readers are referred to Krueger and Casey (2015), Miles et al. (2014), and Tolley et al. (2016) for information on how to collect and analyze qualitative data.

The initial output of qualitative formative evaluation is a transcript that documents what was said verbatim or only slightly edited to remove conversational distractors. The intervention team will need to translate and reduce this text, organizing and presenting the information shared so that it is accessible and meaningful to others. This translational step is often referred to as *thematic analysis*, where the raw transcript is reviewed looking for themes. For the purpose of designing an intervention, the themes to look for are descriptors or labels for factors or determinants that are influencing a behavioral response. The job of the team analyzing the transcripts is to carefully read and attempt to translate what was said by participants in the interviews or focus groups into determinants. The team's prior experience with the evidence table and examining behavioral theories will be helpful because it provides a context for the information and potential labels for what is expressed.

INSIGHTS FOR INTERVENTIONISTS: WHO TO TALK WITH AND WHAT TO ASK DURING QUALITATIVE FORMATIVE ASSESSMENTS

In this phase of planning, the team is trying to understand the factors that influence the behavior of interest in the population that they are working with. Potential participants for interview and focus groups might include the population that will be directly targeted by the intervention, individuals who may be involved in developing and administering the intervention, and other stakeholders who might have unique insights into how the health issue and the related behavior are experienced in the population of interest. In addition, the team needs to connect with those who are influential in creating the social and physical environments that affect the behavior. Using the example of a school-based intervention to reduce middle school students' consumption of SSBs, the qualitative evaluation might be conducted with students, parents, teachers, school food service personnel, and administrators.

Ideally, both focus groups and interviews are conducted. For some stakeholders, the team might want more specific and detailed information, making an interview more efficient. Other times, the team might want to stimulate a broader discussion of issues, making focus groups the preferred method of data collection. Considering the example of an intervention to reduce SSB consumption, individual interviews with the administrators and food service staff who are responsible for setting school-level policy and for making SSBs available at school will likely provide more useful information than combining stakeholders into a focus group. On the other hand, conducting focus groups with students and teachers might provide a richer understanding of the issues regarding student and teacher consumption of SSBs and their real and perceived exposure to SSBs during the school day.

Both interviews and focus groups will require the development of an interview guide that includes a set of questions to ask (Tolley et al., 2016). Questions should be open-ended and provide enough context to ensure that participants are able to respond. Questions should focus on understanding the determinants at the physical, social, and individual levels that may influence behavior. They may be designed to learn whether determinants for the behavior identified through the literature search or suggested by theory apply to the target population and, if so, how. At the same time, questions should be broad enough to allow for new determinants to emerge. Creating opportunities and space during interviews and focus groups to hear the unexpected is essential.

Table 3.5 includes examples of how direct quotes from a focus group with students about what influences their choice of beverages at school and at home are translated into determinants. Notice that determinants can represent barriers as well as facilitators of behavior; for example, not knowing that lemonade and energy drinks are SSBs represents a lack of knowledge. Also, distinctions may be made between actual and perceived barriers reported in qualitative research. For example, the belief heard from the focus groups that "soft drinks are available at home because of water quality and cost" may be translated into "there is a perception that tap water quality is not good and that soft drinks are cheaper than bottled water." Because these barriers may be both real and perceived, determinants related to barriers may be included at both the individual and physical environment levels.

At the completion of the formative evaluation phase, the team should create a list of all of the determinants of the behavior suggested by their (a) evidence table, (b) review of potentially useful theoretical constructs, and (c) formative evaluation. The list of determinants should be organized by the individual, social, and physical environments.

Choosing Relevant Determinants for the Intervention Focus

From this list of determinants, the intervention team will need to choose a set of determinants that will be the focus of the intervention. The goal will be to identify about six to eight determinants expected to have the greatest chance of high impact change on the target behavior. To successfully change a determinant is exceptionally challenging and often involves multiple intervention components. Therefore, it is important to choose a limited number of determinants so that appropriate attention, time, and resources can be allocated to intervention efforts (Perry, 1999).

TABLE 3.5. Translating Qualitative Information Into Determinants: Example From the Healthy Teens/Healthy Planet Intervention to Reduce the Intake of Sugar-Sweetened Beverages (SSBs)

Sample quote from student focus groups	Determinant (environmental level)
"I just drink lemonade and energy drinks; I never drink soda pop."	Lack of knowledge (individual environment)
"Soft drinks are available in vending machines at school but only at certain hours. Our teachers drink soda during class, though."	Availability (physical environment) Observational learning (social environment)
"My parents don't trust that our tap water at home is safe, so we buy bottled soft drinks. Soft drinks are cheaper than bottled water."	Barriers, accessibility (water quality; cost of bottled water) Barriers, perceptions of accessibility (perceptions of water quality and cost)
"I like the taste of soft drinks—water is boring."	Barriers, habits, preferences (individual environment)

The determinants chosen should represent at least two of the three environmental levels from the design framework (individual, social, and physical environments; see Chapter 1). Working on at least two environmental levels increases the chances that the intervention will have a greater impact, that change will be maintained in individuals and organizations participating in the program, and that the program will be disseminated more broadly. Although determinants likely have been identified at the macrolevel throughout this planning process (e.g., urban/rural differences or average level of education in a community), the intervention's ability to change those determinants in a

INSIGHT FOR INTERVENTIONISTS: KEY CONSIDERATIONS FOR CHOOSING THE DETERMINANTS FOR THE FOCUS OF THE INTERVENTION

- What determinants emerged as the best candidates based on the empirical research and scoring the evidence table?

- What determinants emerged as important through the formative work in the community? Do they map onto any determinants also found in the literature?

- Are there determinants that were informed by theory that the team should consider, even if they didn't come up in the empirical literature or in the formative work?

- How strong is the relationship between the behavior and the determinant as evidenced through the empirical research, theory, and formative work?

- How changeable or mutable is the determinant in the targeted population group?

- Was there any evidence of other intervention studies being successful in changing the determinant? Are there elements of those interventions that the team can adapt?

- Considering resources (personnel, money, and time), what determinants can most realistically be changed by this team, at this time, in this community, and with the resources available?

- Considering the community partners that will be involved in the project, are there some determinants from the social or physical environments that would complement their work and missions?

- Are there some determinants that represent "low-hanging fruit"—that is, determinants that could be changed with relative ease and timeliness? Even if the potential impact of change in that determinant may be relatively low, it may be important to show stakeholders that progress was made and some success experienced. Small successes may help fuel (and fund) initiatives to tackle bigger challenges.

time-limited intervention study or community program is unlikely. Determinants from the macrolevel will not be included as potential determinants to change with the intervention, but they must be considered as the team enters the next phase of creating the intervention. These macrolevel determinants may be considered in analyses as covariates or as moderators of the effects of the intervention on the targeted outcomes during the Evaluate Phase.

Example of Choosing Determinants: Healthy Teens, Healthy Planet

Let's look back at the task of identifying the determinants for school-based intervention to reduce the SSB intake of adolescents. Using the evidence table and the scoring exercise that the team completed (Table 3.4), the following determinants scored the highest:

- **Perceived behavioral control:** Increase students' self-efficacy about their ability to make healthier beverage choices

- **Perceived barriers:** Change habits and influence preferences; change perceptions about the price of water versus SSBs

- **Descriptive norms:** Change perceptions about peers' SSB preferences

- **Availability of beverages at school:** Positively influence beverage options available in vending machines and other venues; positively influence bottled water pricing

A look at theory and an understanding of the population suggests that the social and physical environment is likely important, so the team considers adding the following items to the list of potential determinants:

- **Observational learning:** Impact the social environment so that healthy beverage choices are modeled

- **Social reinforcements:** Change social reinforcements so that the healthy choice is reinforced

Finally, the qualitative formative research suggested that the following determinants should be considered:

- **Knowledge:** Improve knowledge about which beverages count as SSBs

- **Teachers' behaviors:** Work on school policies to reduce teachers' consumption of SSBs in class

- **Availability and price of beverage choices at school:** Work with schools to reduce the cost of water relative to the cost of SSBs and reduce the availability of SSBs in the school

The determinant regarding availability and accessibility of beverages at school came up twice, through the empirical research and the formative research. Therefore, eight determinants were identified as the focus of the intervention: three from the individual environment (perceived control, perceived barriers, knowledge); three from the social environment (descriptive norms, observational learning, social reinforcement); and two from the physical environment (availability; relative price of SSBs). The team feels good about these determinants: They represent multiple environmental levels, there was good evidence that the chosen determinants are important in their population, and the team can envision potential and realistic intervention channels and approaches.

STEP 3: CREATE A CONCEPTUAL MODEL

After the set of determinants to be targeted is finalized, the team is ready to produce the conceptual model. The conceptual model acts as the blueprint for guiding the rest of the intervention design process and provides a clear statement of where the project is headed for all relevant stakeholders. It clarifies the factors that will be the focus of the intervention for community stakeholders and shows the evaluation team the determinants, behaviors, and other variables that will need to be assessed.

What Is a Conceptual Model?

In general, a *conceptual model* is a graphic representation of the proposed causal linkages among a set of concepts or constructs related to an outcome, in this case, a health behavior (Earp & Ennett, 1991). Conceptual models are not the same as theories or larger frameworks such as a social ecological model. Conceptual models focus on hypothesized relationships between a specified health behavior and determinants of that behavior in a targeted population. They do not attempt to account for all of the potential factors that may help explain variability in the behavior. Attention to parsimony is a significant challenge in creating conceptual models. The tendency is to want to include all of the factors that influence a behavioral outcome, including social determinants of health and other factors from the macro environment that are known to have a significant influence on behavior and health. The purpose of creating a conceptual model, however, is to identify a set of potential targets for the intervention and generate hypotheses about how the intervention will work.

Conceptual models are useful in showing determinants across multiple levels of influence and how those levels may interact with each other to influence the outcome (Earp & Ennett, 1991). The general framework for MLIs that was introduced in Chapter 1 of this volume is used as a template for the conceptual model (showing factors in the individual, social, and physical environments interacting with each other and predicting a health behavior), but detail is added to the determinants identified within each environment. In developing a conceptual model, the behavioral outcome is included in a box to the far right and the determinants to be changed, organized by environmental level, are included to the left of the outcome. A box is included to the lower right of the model that suggests potential modifying factors or covariates to be considered in the intervention planning and evaluation. These modifying factors

FIGURE 3.1. Specific Aim and Conceptual Model: Example From the Healthy Teens/Healthy Planet Intervention to Reduce Students' Intake of Sugar-Sweetened Beverages (SSBs)

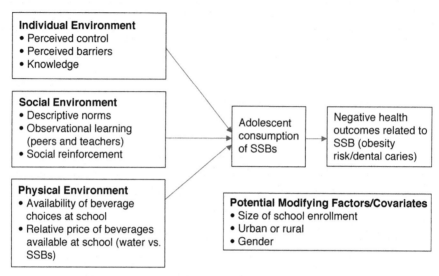

Note. Specific aim: The intervention will reduce students' daily mean consumption of sugar sweetened beverages by 50% of baseline consumption.

or covariates are not in the causal pathway but may impact the relationship between the independent and dependent variables or be confounding variables. For now, showing simple relationships of constructs within the model will suffice; later, as the evaluation plan is furthered developed, more detail can be added, suggesting relationships to test and potential moderators to examine. The conceptual model also includes a heading that states the specific aim of the intervention, including the behavior to be changed and the population targeted. Sometimes the degree of expected change in the behavior (also called the "primary outcome" for the evaluation work) is included in the specific aim.

Example Conceptual Model: Healthy Teens, Healthy Planet

Figure 3.1 shows an example of a conceptual model and its specific aim, using the example of creating a school-based intervention to reduce the consumption of SSB. The model shows the eight determinants that have been chosen as the focus of the intervention activities organized by environment and suggests a causal relationship between the determinants and adolescent consumption of SSBs as well as the behavior's link to important health-related outcomes: obesity risk and dental caries. The model also includes several modifying factors and covariates that will be considered as the intervention is developed and evaluated including two factors at the school level (size of school district and if the school is in an urban or rural area) as well as the gender of the students participating in the intervention and measurement activities.

STEP 4: REVIEW THE CONCEPTUAL MODEL WITH THE EVALUATION TEAM AND COMMUNITY STAKEHOLDERS

Typically, the individuals responsible for creating the intervention are a different group of individuals than those responsible for the evaluation of the project. This division of labor happens for a number of reasons, including the different skill sets that are required for each task and the need to divide the work to ensure that timelines are met. When conducting a rigorous evaluation of an intervention, those individuals who collect data should not be the same as those who have interacted with participants as part of intervention activities. This separation is necessary to minimize response bias.

Communication between the intervention and evaluation teams is essential throughout the process but particularly during the Plan Phase as elements of the intervention development and evaluation planning happen in tandem. As the intervention team moves on to creating the intervention, the evaluation team will need to make decisions about the best study design and the measures to be collected to test the specific aim and hypothesis. The intervention and evaluation team will review the conceptual model together to clarify the specific aim and hypothesis to be tested in the intervention trial or program evaluation as well as the primary outcome, determinants, and covariates to be assessed. The *primary outcome* is the behavior that the intervention will attempt to change and must be measurable (meaning that a valid and reliable measurement tool to assess the outcome is available or can be developed within the study's timeframe), and change must be reasonable to expect within the timeline of the study.

In addition to having a robust measurement tool for the behavior they hope to change, the team will also want to be able to evaluate change in the determinants; intervention strategies will be designed and delivered with the intent of changing determinants. If the intervention is not successful in making a positive impact on determinants, it is unlikely that behavior change will be achieved. Determinants to be measured will include those from the individual environment (e.g., knowledge and attitudes), the social environment (e.g., the presence of social cues in the environment), and the physical environment (e.g., measures of availability and accessibility in the physical environment). Determinants may be evaluated as secondary outcomes or as mediators.

Other measurement needs to consider include those factors that may affect the relationship between the determinants and the behavior. Sometimes these factors are used as moderators or covariates in the analysis. Moderators and covariates may include immutable determinants, such as age, race/ethnicity, or education or may include mutable factors that were not targeted by the intervention but may explain how individuals responded to the intervention, such as perceived self-efficacy or level of awareness. Moderation allows an examination of the possibility that the relationship between the determinants and the outcome differ by subgroups (e.g., males compared with females or younger people compared with older people). Sometimes the factors that may affect the relationship between the determinants and behavior are included as covariates in an analytic model where their potential impact is controlled for analytically. Measurement issues are discussed in more detail in the Evaluate Phase (see Chapter 6). Communication with community-level stakeholders is an important part of this final step in the Plan Phase. A review of the conceptual model, along with an explanation of how decisions were made, should be shared with relevant community stakeholders. In addition, this is a good time to share information on the next steps in the process, allowing stakeholders the opportunity to provide additional feedback on the current plans.

Developing the Intervention Manual of Procedures

Finally, this is the time in the design process to begin to pull together information for an intervention manual of procedures (IMOP). The purpose of the IMOP is to describe and document the intervention. In this document, the "black box" of the intervention is unpacked to provide details regarding all aspects of the intervention, including what was delivered, for whom, how delivery occurred, and how frequently. The IMOP is the crucial source of information regarding the intervention and is used to document the myriad decisions the intervention team makes during the entire intervention design process. It is used to orient new members of the project team and new stakeholders who become involved with the project throughout the intervention. As intervention trials and program initiatives ramp up, staffing and stakeholders often change; to have a single source document with details of the intervention creates important efficiency for the team. Assembly of the IMOP begins during the Plan Phase and grows as details of the intervention are finalized. It exists as a draft document and is not "final" until the intervention is complete. It then serves as the complete description of the intervention as planned, with all details archived in one document.

Exhibit 3.2 describes all of the information that will ultimately be included in the IMOP. For the Plan Phase, the IMOP will include the first four items of the overview including a general description of the overall goal of the intervention and related outcomes, the environmental levels that will be targeted by the intervention, a description of community engagement activities, and the conceptual model that is produced in this Plan Phase. Details about the intervention and community engagement will be expanded upon as the intervention design process progresses.

Creating an IMOP may seem like a great deal of work, but in many ways it simply involves documenting decisions and organizing materials that evolve as the team plans, creates, implements, and evaluates an intervention. In addition, the materials compiled and created for the IMOP often serve multiple purposes. As an example, the overview summarizes the intervention and states how it will work to achieve the study's primary outcome. It includes a description of the levels targeted through the intervention and community engagement in the

EXHIBIT 3.2

Information to be Included in the Intervention Manual of Procedures

- An overview that includes the following:
    1. a paragraph or two describing the overall goal of the intervention and primary and secondary outcomes
    2. a paragraph or two describing each environmental level of the intervention and how the levels work together to create a single intervention or program
    3. a description of community engagement activities
    4. the conceptual model guiding the intervention showing the determinants the intervention will focus on to effect behavior change
    5. the intervention logic model
    6. a table showing the intervention objectives, corresponding intervention strategies, and intervention components
    7. a timeline for intervention activities
    8. descriptions of how intervention participants at each level were identified and recruited for participation
- For each environmental level, the following are included:
    1. descriptions of how each intervention component is implemented, including timing, dose, who delivers the intervention strategy, and materials needed
    2. details on what occurs at each session or each contact point with participants
    3. copies of all materials produced (including written materials, text messages, Internet-based materials including website content and posts and content for social media, scripts for interventionists)
    4. other level-specific protocol and correspondence
- Activities related to standardizing the intervention include the following:
    1. training needs, protocol, and related materials
    2. communication process for intervention team (e.g., plans for providing rapid feedback on the intervention, fidelity checks, retraining needs)
- Plans for collecting process data and the related process forms, including assessing fidelity of the intervention delivery, the reach of the intervention, and the dose received by participants
- Any changes in protocol as the intervention proceeds

process. Such a summary will be useful for a variety of purposes, including describing the project to community stakeholders or the intervention for research purposes. Likewise, a plethora of decisions are documented in the IMOP, including decisions related to the timing of the intervention, decisions about the intervention strategies and components to be used, and decisions about how to recruit and retain individuals and groups to participate in the intervention. As such, the IMOP serves as the institutional memory of the decisions made about the intervention. The IMOP should be saved as a digital file and updated regularly, clearly documenting and dating the current version.

SUMMARY OF THE PLAN PHASE

The Plan Phase starts with making sure that the team has identified a behavior-based health problem that is appropriate for a multilevel community intervention. The next step of this phase involves going through the process of reviewing relevant behavior change theory, examining the existing literature, and hearing the voices of the community stakeholders to understand the determinants, or influences, of the behavior. The phase continues with choosing a set of determinants on which to intervene and creating a conceptual model that serves as the blueprint for both intervention and evaluation activities. Early in the process community stakeholders are engaged in identifying a health issue of concern to the community and, through formative assessment, provide their opinions about how the community experiences the behavior and the factors in their community that influence it. This phase ends with reviewing the conceptual model with stakeholders and the evaluation team.

Without carefully progressing through these steps of the Plan Phase, the entire project is threatened. Many other forces will pull on both research and practitioner teams working on health behavior change in a community setting. Some of these forces may include deadlines that prevent adequate time for identifying determinants and environmental levels to focus on or insufficient time to look for interventions to adapt. Other forces that may threaten the planning process are specific interests of stakeholders who want to use an intervention that has not been carefully developed. In addition, there is a tendency to prioritize time, attention, and money for the evaluation and analytic needs of the project over intervention needs. But without a strong intervention, it is unlikely that significant results will be found regardless of how sophisticated the evaluation approach. The steps of the Plan Phase help the team focus on the goal of the intervention, feel confident that they have made good decisions about its focus, and provide a strong rationale to others for the decisions they have made.

4

The Create Phase

The second phase of the design process is the Create Phase. In this phase, the intervention team uses all of the information obtained and decisions made in the Plan Phase to create the intervention. This chapter starts with an explanation of terms used in this volume to describe parts of the intervention and then turns to information on writing intervention objectives and deciding on the intervention components to use (Step 5). This step includes a discussion about some of the advantages and limitations of environment-specific components. Step 6 involves designing the specific intervention strategies within each component to meet intervention objectives. In addition, suggestions on how to assemble a creative team and examples of how to integrate approaches from change theories to adapt or create new intervention strategies are included in this step. The next step, Step 7, create a logic model, provides detail on the resources needed to implement the intervention. The final step in the Create Phase (Step 8) is to share intervention plans and the logic model with both community stakeholders and members of the evaluation team. Throughout this phase, the hypothetical "Healthy Teens, Healthy Planet" school-based intervention is used as an exemplar for showing how intervention components and strategies are developed. A logic model for the "Healthy Teens, Healthy Planet" intervention is included.

https://doi.org/10.1037/0000292-005
Designing Interventions to Promote Community Health: A Multilevel, Stepwise Approach, by L. A. Lytle

The steps included in the Create Phase are as follows:

5. Write the intervention objectives and identify potential intervention components
6. Design intervention strategies
7. Create a logic model
8. Share the logic model with the evaluation team and community stakeholders

STEP 5: WRITE THE INTERVENTION OBJECTIVES AND IDENTIFY POTENTIAL INTERVENTION COMPONENTS

The first step of the Create Phase is to write intervention objectives that correspond to the previously identified determinants and identify appropriate intervention components. In this book, I make distinctions between different aspects of interventions, including intervention objectives, components, strategies, and techniques:

- An *intervention objective* is a simple statement that describes how each determinant will be changed by the intervention; it is only declarative in nature and does not provide any sense of how the intervention will work to create that change.

- An *intervention component* is a broad approach that describes the general mechanism by which the intervention objectives will be met. For example, a classroom curriculum, a digitally delivered social support program, a social media campaign, or a policy approach to change the physical environment are examples of intervention components. Multilevel interventions (MLIs) typically contain more than one intervention component.

DISTINCTIONS BETWEEN ASPECTS OF INTERVENTIONS

- **Intervention objective:** A statement that describes how the determinant will be changed by the intervention

- **Intervention component:** The broader approaches to be used to meet intervention objectives

- **Intervention strategies:** The specific activities, messages, and related materials used within each intervention component to meet intervention objectives

- **Intervention techniques:** Specific techniques from behavior change theory used to help instigate change in an intervention

- *Intervention strategies* are the specific activities that are used within each component to meet intervention objectives. For example, for a classroom curricular component, the individual lessons, related materials, and the plans for how often the lessons are delivered and by whom make up the specific intervention strategies. For a social media campaign, the messages, scripts, promotional materials, and plans for the timing and duration of messaging and outreach make up the specific intervention strategies. Intervention strategies are what makes an intervention unique.

- Finally, *intervention techniques* are specific techniques from behavior change theory that are used to help instigate change. For example, lessons (intervention strategies) from the classroom curricula (intervention component) may include skills training and reinforcements (behavior change techniques) as a way to help students build skills related to preparing a healthy snack.

Writing Intervention Objectives

The intervention objectives describe how the determinants related to the health behavior will be changed by the program. Intervention objectives can be positively or negatively worded, and each determinant should be the focus of one or more objectives. Multiple intervention objectives addressing a single determinant point to the importance of the determinant, suggesting that change will be attempted through several approaches and more resources will be allocated to changing the determinant (Perry, 1999). Intervention objectives are not the same as a specific aim; they do not describe how the behavioral outcome is expected to change based on the intervention. Rather, they state how the intervention will affect each behavioral determinant.

Table 4.1 uses the example of a hypothetical school-based intervention to reduce student consumption of sugar-sweetened beverages (SSBs) to show how intervention objectives are written for each determinant. (As noted in Chapter 3 of this volume, the name Healthy Teens, Healthy Planet is not established by the intervention team until Step 6 of this phase.) For each determinant, at least one corresponding intervention objective is presented that describes what the intervention will do to have a positive impact on the determinant. As an example, to positively affect student-level perceived control of their SSB intake, the intervention will specifically work to "increase students' confidence that they can make healthier beverage choices while at school" and will also "enhance students' skills in being able to choose beverages without added sugar." The specification included in the intervention objective reflects what was learned about how the determinant is related to the behavior during the formative assessment in the Plan Phase. As another example, the determinant from the physical environment, "Relative price of beverages available," will specifically be addressed in the intervention through objectives to "decrease the price of bottled water relative to the price of SSB" and "make available and promote the use of water dispensers throughout the school."

Note that by organizing the determinants and corresponding intervention objectives by each of the three environmental levels, an MLI is being built.

TABLE 4.1. Writing Intervention Objectives for Each Determinant: Example From Healthy Teens, Healthy Planet

Determinant	Intervention objective
Individual environment	
Perceived control	Increase students' *confidence* that they can make healthier beverage choices while at school
	Enhance students' *skills* in being able to choose beverages without added sugar
Perceived barriers	Increase students' *perceptions* that healthy beverage choices are socially positive
	Increase students' *awareness* of price comparisons among SSBs, bottled water, and water dispensers in school
	Increase students' *acceptance* of using water bottles and water dispensers available in school
Knowledge	Increase students' *knowledge* of what types of beverages include added sugar
	Increase students' *knowledge* about the healthfulness of water compared with SSBs
Social environment	
Observational learning/ role modeling	Decrease *exposure* to students and school staff drinking SSBs
	Increase *exposure* to students and staff choosing water as a beverage
Descriptive norm	Increase *shared social experience* that many adolescents prefer water as a beverage
Social reinforcement	Increase *reinforcement* of choosing water over SSBs
Physical environment	
Availability of beverage choices at school	Work with school administration and staff to reduce the *availability* of SSBs on the school property
	Work with school administration and staff to increase the *accessibility* of water on the school property
Relative price of beverages available	Work with school administration to *decrease the price of* bottled water relative to the price of SSBs
	Work with school administration to *make available and promote* the use of water dispensers throughout the school

Note. SSBs = sugar-sweetened beverages.

At the individual environment, the objectives focus on changing student-level factors related to beverage choice, including student confidence, skills, perceptions, awareness, acceptance, and knowledge. Intervention objectives from the social environment focus on changing what students are exposed to and observe during the school day and how beverage-related behavior is modeled by both students and staff. This observational learning or role-modeling has the potential to influence descriptive norms related to the social behaviors experienced by the students as well as what they observe about social reinforcements that others receive by making healthy beverage choices. Finally, to change the determinants related to the physical environment, the intervention will include work with school change agents to positively influence the availability, accessibility, and environmental cueing of behaviors. Intervention goals will focus on making water more available and SSBs less available in schools and improving accessibility by making water more affordable relative to the cost of SSBs. Environmental cues and promotions will encourage students' use of water dispensers throughout the school.

The simple structure of an intervention objective allows others, including the target group and other community-level stakeholders, to understand how the intervention will work to positively affect each determinant identified in the Plan Phase. This simplicity is important for clarity of communication and transparency of intent. As the intervention objectives are shared with others, another opportunity to engage the community opens up. Stakeholders stay informed, support from the community can be garnered, and the intervention developers can confirm that the intervention plans are on track to be relevant and meaningful to stakeholders.

Identifying Potential Interventions Components

Although the intervention objectives state how the intervention will affect the determinant, they do not include any detail on how that change will be achieved. Finalizing decisions about the intervention objectives involves a consideration of the broader approaches to create change, referred to as the intervention components. To a large extent, intervention components map onto approaches that specifically target the individual, social, or physical environment, although many components may affect multiple environments. Table 4.2 shows a list of potential intervention components and the environments where they may be useful, highlighting in bold the environment most directly affected by the component.

Intervention components focusing on changing determinants from the individual environment include the use of classes, curricula, individual or group counseling, and health communication designed to connect directly with an individual to influence knowledge, build skills, change beliefs, or motivate. These approaches may be delivered face-to-face, through online classes, through print material, or using digital approaches such as emails or text messages.

Intervention components that are most effective in changing determinants from the social environment include programs that attempt to increase peer or social support, impact social networks, and influence social cognitions. They may include social marketing or media campaigns focusing on changing norms as well as policy and practice changes that influence the social experience around a health behavior. Digital interventions designed to encourage and enhance social support through chat rooms and creating online supportive social networks are examples of intervention components targeting the social environment. Intervention components targeting the social environment may directly involve members of the social group to deliver aspects of the intervention. A community health model in which peer leaders help deliver aspects of the

TABLE 4.2. Examples of Intervention Components and the Environments They Impact

Intervention component	Individual environment	Social environment	Physical environment
Curriculum/classes (in-person, online)	**X**	X	
One-on-one counseling (in-person, remote, online)	**X**		
Group counseling (in-person, remote, online)	**X**	X	
Health communication (print, media)	**X**		
Media campaign	X	**X**	
Social marketing campaign	X	**X**	
Educational drama	X	X	
Developing social/peer support	X	**X**	
Enhancing and engaging social networks	X	**X**	
Use of peer leaders	X	**X**	
Use of community health workers	X	**X**	
Policies and practices to change the social environment	X	**X**	
Policies and practices to change physical environment	X	X	**X**
Change in the built environment	X	X	**X**
Taxation and price promotions	X	X	**X**
Health messages and cues in the environment	X	X	**X**

Note. X in bold represents the environment most directly affected by the component.

intervention is an example of a component that is especially effective in influencing the social environment (Fisher et al., 2015).

Intervention components that focus on changing determinants from the physical environment are those designed to create change in the physical space. These changes may involve restricting the availability of certain products or behavioral options by enacting a policy (e.g., prohibiting smoking) or changing behavioral opportunities in an environment (e.g., eliminating cigarette vending machines). Intervention components designed to affect the physical environment may also include messages in the environment to inform or cue behavior (e.g., food labels, promotional signs) or use fear arousal to discourage a behavior (e.g., warning labels on cigarette packages). Components targeting the physical environment might also include financial incentives and price promotions that improve accessibility.

While a component may largely map onto an approach that specifically targets the individual, social, or physical environment, most will have an impact on multiple environments. For example, although a class or group counseling session may provide information and skill building with a focus on changing the behavior of individuals in class, being part of a group may also have an impact on one's social environment. The leader of the group may provide social support or encouragement to each individual, and the content of the class or counseling session may include activities to encourage group support among participants. Likewise, when behavioral options change in the physical environment, people's social and individual environments likely change as well. For example, the addition of walking paths for employees on site positively changes the physical environment of the worksite. As the opportunities to walk increase, more workers choose to walk at breaks and become positive role models for other workers. Eventually, walking at breaks becomes "what we do at work," changing social expectations and norms. When individuals see coworkers add physical activity to their workday, their own self-efficacy for being able to make that change may be enhanced. Intervention components that have potential to change determinants at multiple levels simultaneously may provide efficiency and increase the potential for and potency of change.

Intervention components may be chosen based on their record of success observed in general practice or identified in the literature. The literature review done as part of the Plan Phase may have revealed effective interventions targeting the same behavior in similar communities. Examining the intervention components that they used will provide important insights into ways to achieve intervention objectives. Intervention components are also chosen based on their acceptability to the community and the feasibility of implementing the intervention approach including costs and other resources. Importantly, intervention components are chosen based on the anticipated potency that they will have in meeting the intervention objective (Perry, 1999). Resources are always limited, and thus, choosing components that have the best chance to deliver strong intervention strategies is crucial.

Example of Choosing Intervention Components: Healthy Teens, Healthy Planet

Circling back to the example being developed for designing a school-based intervention to reduce student consumption of SSBs, for this step in the intervention design process, the intervention team would review the intervention objectives and decide on the most potent and feasible intervention component to use to meet those objectives. Based on what they learned from the review of the literature, their formative assessment and considering their resources, budget, and timeline, the team decides that they will use three intervention components: (a) a classroom curriculum with peer-led elements, (b) a school-wide social marketing campaign, and (c) policy and practice approaches. The classroom curriculum will be used as the primary vehicle to influence students' perceived control, perceived barriers, and knowledge. A curricular approach is particularly well suited to building student confidence in their ability to make healthier choices through lessons focusing on practicing behavioral skills on how to make healthier beverages choices

ADVANTAGES AND LIMITATIONS OF ENVIRONMENT-SPECIFIC COMPONENTS

Components With a Focus on the Individual Environment
Advantages

- Ability to create tailored approaches and messages that speak directly to an individual's situation
- Ability to provide reinforcements that are valued by the individual
- Ability to provide direct social support and encouragement

Limitations

- Rarely results in long-term, sustained change without supporting components
- Reach is limited; individuals must "sign up" and consistently "show up"
- Cost of providing individualized or group intervention is expensive and typically recurring

Components With a Focus on the Social Environment
Advantages

- Good evidence that many health behaviors are "contagious," or spread through social groups (Christakis & Fowler, 2007)
- Good evidence that changing social norms is an effective way to change behavior (Fell & Voas, 2006)
- Potential for widespread and durable impact

Limitations

- Need to identify the social referents most important to the behavior to be changed
- Many social influences exist in the broader social and cultural environment
- May require social referents to provide active social support

Components With a Focus on the Physical Environment
Advantages

- Individuals become passive recipients and can be "nudged" toward the healthy behavior (Thaler & Sunstein, 2008)
- Reach is large; all of those interacting with the environment are affected regardless of their personal interests in behavior change
- Increased chance for sustainability of behavior and system change

Limitations

- "Big P" policy changes with a focus on legislative or large, system-wide change take a long time to enact
- May require a substantial cost and commitment (i.e., adding sidewalks to a neighborhood or bringing in a full-service grocery store to a food desert)

(e.g., reading labels). In addition, curricular activities can be developed to change awareness of price comparisons between beverage choices at school and to increase student knowledge about why water is a healthy choice. The use of peer leaders in the delivery of some of the intervention activities will help promote positive role modeling (part of the social environment) while also help to increase perceived control, reduce barriers, and increase knowledge. The use of a health curriculum to positively impact the individual environment is a well-established practice that has been shown to be effective in changing students' beliefs and motivations. The intervention team will need to include teachers and school administration as they begin to plan out the details of the intervention strategies to be used in this component.

The primary component used to have an impact on the social environment will be a social marketing campaign that will attempt to change descriptive norms and emphasize the social benefits of choosing water over SSBs. This component may include postings on the school's Facebook page, posters, and mini dramas performed by students as part of the school announcements. The specific intervention strategies (including messages to promote and visuals to use) will need to be developed with input from students, but a member of the team has experience in designing marketing campaigns, and the team is confident that this component will be effective in influencing the social environment.

The final component is a policy and practice approach, working with school leaders to have an impact on both the social and physical environments of school. The concept of a healthy school environment has been promoted by the Centers for Disease Control and Prevention (CDC) for decades (https://www. cdc.gov/healthyschools/). Approaches to achieve the related intervention objectives might include working toward policy and practice change to impact the beverage choices of important referents in the school environment (both peers and school staff). In addition, the policy and practice component will move toward limiting, and ultimately eliminating, the availability of SSBs on the school grounds while increasing the availability of water dispensers throughout the school. Table 4.3 shows how the components match up with the determinants and intervention objectives.

Notice that some of the components do double duty by making an impact on multiple intervention objectives simultaneously. For example, the peer-led curriculum component will affect determinants from both individual and social environments through the use of peer leaders as role models. The social marketing campaign may include a media campaign showing students drinking water and using reusable water bottles at dispensing stations at school. This component will work to influence perceived barriers at the individual level and descriptive norms at the social environmental level. Students' acceptance of using the water dispensing stations throughout the school brought about by the policy and practice component can be fostered through the information provided in the school curriculum as well as the social marketing campaign showing that other students choose water over SSBs. The degree to which the components work synergistically increases both the potency of change from the intervention and its efficiency.

TABLE 4.3. Identifying Intervention Components: Example From the Healthy Teens/Healthy Planet Intervention to Reduce the Intake of Sugar-Sweetened Beverages (SSBs)

Component	Determinant	Intervention objective
Individual environment		
Classroom curriculum	Perceived control	Increase students' *confidence* that they can make healthier beverage choices while at school
		Enhance students' *skills* in being able to choose beverages without added sugar
Classroom curriculum	Perceived barriers	Increase students' *perceptions* that healthy beverage choices are socially positive
		Increase students' *awareness* of price comparisons between SSBs, bottled water, and water dispensers in school
		Increase students' *acceptance* of using water bottles and water dispensers available in school
Classroom curriculum	Knowledge	Increase students' *knowledge* of what types of beverages include added sugar
		Increase students' *knowledge* about the healthfulness of water as compared with SSBs
Social environment		
Social media campaign	Role modeling	Decrease *exposure* to students and school staff drinking SSBs
Classroom curriculum (through peer lead activities)		Increase *exposure* to students and staff choosing water as a beverage
Policies and practices		
Social media campaign	Descriptive norm	Increase *beliefs* that many adolescents prefer water as a beverage
Policies and practices		
Social media campaign	Social reinforcement	Increase *reinforcement* of choosing water over SSBs
Policies and practices		
Physical environment		
Policies and practices	Availability of beverage choices at school	Work with school officials and staff to reduce the *availability* of SSBs on the school property
		Work with school officials and staff to increase the *accessibility* of water on the school property
Policies and practices	Relative price of beverages available	Work with school officials to *decrease the price of* bottled water relative to the price of SSBs
		Work with school officials to *make available and promote* water dispensers throughout the school

After the intervention components are decided upon, many details will need to be worked out. For example, for the school curriculum, the team will need to work with school administrators, curriculum specialists, and classroom teachers to figure out the following: What educational competencies will be met through the lessons? How many lessons should be planned, and how much class time is available for delivering the lessons? What types of kitchen facilities might be needed for food-related activities? Who will deliver the lessons—project staff or classroom teachers?

The social marketing campaign will need to be developed in close collaboration with students, school staff, and school administration. The messages and approaches for the social marketing campaign need to be relevant and appropriate for the audience and capture how the determinants of the behavior are represented in the school. The intervention team will need to see what other types of social media the school uses and whether there are ways to complement what they are already doing. For the policy and practice approaches, the team will need to consider how the school goes about creating or changing policy and practice. Is there a process that they will need to follow, or will they need to develop a new way to create policy and practice change? Is there an existing school wellness committee that works on policy and practice issues? School administration and other school-level influencers (including teachers, other staff, parents, and students) will need to be involved.

STEP 6: DESIGN INTERVENTION STRATEGIES

Now that the team has identified the determinants that the intervention will attempt to change, written the intervention objectives, and decided on the components that the team will use to deliver the intervention, they are ready to begin creating the intervention strategies. These are the specific activities, messages, and related materials that will make this intervention unique. Think of the conceptual model created in the Plan Phase as the blueprint for a house (i.e., How big will the house be? How many floors? How is the house situated on the property?). Choosing the components to be used to deliver the intervention adds the walls and windows and determines the flow through the house. Designing the intervention strategies gets down to the details that make the house unique (i.e., What color do we paint the walls? What material do we put on the floors? What lighting fixtures and appliances should we choose?). As such, this is one of the most fun and creative parts of designing an intervention.

Although this step is very creative, all of the previous planning work needs to stay in the forefront of the design process. The groundwork done identifying the determinants of the behavior, writing intervention objectives, and deciding on the appropriate intervention components provides the structure for the development of the intervention strategies. Without this structure, team members may build an intervention that appeals to their creativity but strays from the objectives of the intervention. It takes a special team to create the intervention strategies.

INSIGHTS FOR INTERVENTIONISTS: BUILDING THE CREATIVE TEAM

The step of designing intervention strategies requires as much art as science. There is no single source for intervention strategies; no catalog of activities to pick and choose from. Therefore, the team members involved with this step need to include creative people who know how to grab the attention of and engage the target audience. Creative people provide humor, relevance, and life to a health behavior program and have the skills necessary to communicate with people in ways that many health professionals may lack. In identifying creative people to be on the intervention design team, look for those who have been involved in creative endeavors before, have designed and implemented interventions using the intervention components that have been chosen for the current project, and have some experience working with the target audience.

In addition to creative-types, the team working on developing the intervention strategies needs to include community-based stakeholders. Directly involving at least one community member in planning intervention strategies helps ensure that the activities chosen are relevant to community needs and that intervention approaches are feasible to deliver in the community.

Programs that include community input during their creation increase their chances that other community stakeholders will be supportive of the intervention activities and program at large. This support may be essential in securing the community's short-term commitment to the project and may also increase the chances for program sustainability. Importantly, by directly engaging members from the community in the creative process, community capacity is being built. If possible, hire people from the community to be involved in designing the intervention strategies. At the very least, pay at least one community member to provide regular input as the plans are developed.

Considering Intervention Strategies

Deciding on the intervention strategies to use begins by reviewing what other groups have done to change similar determinants and the strategies that seemed to work well. The literature review done in the Plan Phase may have identified previous interventions that targeted the same determinants; if they were effective, similar intervention strategies may be considered for this new project, saving time, money, and valuable resources. If the team plans to use existing intervention strategies, some adaptation may need to occur to make the approach and materials relevant to the community with which the team is working. Chapter 7 in this volume includes guidelines for adapting interventions as well as sources of evidence-based interventions. Other times, the intervention team will need to develop new strategies using their collective experience, knowledge, and creativity. A review of theories of how behavior change happens (described in Chapter 2) may provide insights into approaches to use in designing strategies.

An important consideration in choosing intervention strategies is to be realistic about the resources that are available to the project. All projects have constraints, and providing more strategies is not necessarily better for meeting intervention objectives. Choose intervention strategies that are considered to have the best potential to change the targeted determinants and that can be implemented with fidelity and replicated with relative ease. In addition, be realistic about the team's skills. Overreaching what the team can pull off leads to missed deadlines, as well as stress and frustration.

This is a good time to meet with community stakeholders to provide an update on the progress of the project, tell them about the intervention components that will be used to deliver the intervention, and describe next steps. This is also a time to engage both the target audience and other stakeholders in additional formative work as a way help make final decisions about the intervention strategies to be used. Formative work can be used as a way to hear how the target audience talks about the topic, including the words and feelings that they bring to the issue. These insights will help make the materials more relevant and alive to the audience. Formative work with other stakeholders can provide important insights into the potential barriers or challenges to be faced with different types of intervention approaches and is an additional way to generate ideas about potential intervention strategies.

Example of Choosing and Creating Intervention Strategies: Healthy Teens, Healthy Planet

This section returns to the hypothetical example of the school-based intervention to reduce students' consumption of SSBs. The section begins by describing the process of reengaging with community stakeholders to get input on intervention strategies to be used to meet intervention objectives and then describes how the intervention team develops strategies for each intervention component. The use of behavioral theory about how change happens is illustrated, and an example of how intervention strategies from evidence-based interventions may be adapted for a new intervention is provided.

Getting Started: Conducting Additional Formative Evaluation With the Community

The intervention components to be used in the Healthy Teens, Healthy Planet intervention include (a) a classroom curriculum with peer-led elements, (b) a school-wide social marketing campaign, and (c) policy and practice approaches. Next, the team needs to decide on the specific intervention strategies to be used in each component to meet the intervention objectives.

Before the team digs into developing details of the intervention, additional formative evaluation will be helpful. Hearing directly from students will help frame messages for the classroom curriculum and the social marketing campaign. It will be important to hear from school staff to get their input on curricular, social media, and policy approaches that might be particularly appealing and relevant from their viewpoints, as well as approaches that might be particularly challenging or disagreeable.

As the team begins this formative phase, additional meetings with school stakeholders may need to occur, especially if school stakeholders have changed. These meetings should be conducted by school leaders as well as those designing the intervention to show stakeholder buy-in for and participation in the project. Information to be presented might include the rationale for working with the school on the issue of student consumption of SSB, the steps and people involved in getting the project to this point, the timeline of activities, and the components that have been chosen to deliver the intervention. The meeting should discuss next steps, including conducting formative work with students and school staff to help design specific elements of the intervention. This meeting may provide a good opportunity to identify key stakeholders to be involved in the next phase of formative assessment.

The formative assessment includes focus groups with students to (a) understand factors that influence beverage choice at school (taste preference, availability, price, environmental concerns), (b) hear students' beliefs and opinions about the importance of making healthy beverage choices, and (c) understand student perspectives on the ways in which the school environment supports or hinders making healthy beverage choices. For example, focus groups with students may include such questions as the following:

- What beverages do you see students, teachers, and staff drinking during the school day?
- How important do you think it is to drink healthy beverages like water instead of SSBs?
- To what extent do you think that your school's environment influences what you drink while at school (during the school day and at afterschool activities)?
- How would you react if your school restricted drinking SSBs at school?
- Tell me about any rules or practices that restrict what beverages school staff and students drink during class time or in the halls.
- To what extent are SSBs used to reward students?
- Tell me about the availability of good-tasting, cold water throughout the day in your school.

Semistructured interviews will be conducted with the principal, the head of school food service, a small sample of teachers, the school nurse, and a representative from physical education or the athletic department. The interviews will be designed to gain school stakeholders' opinions about the need for written policies or improved school practices related to the availability and accessibility of SSBs and water. If policies are already in place, the school stakeholders will be queried about how those policies are enforced in the school. Questions for school staff will include the following:

- To what extent do you think that your school's environment influences what students drink while at school (during the school day and at afterschool activities)?

- What is your opinion about schools restricting SSB consumption at school?

- Tell me about any rules or practices that restrict what beverages school staff and students drink during class time or in the halls.

- To what extent are SSBs used to provide incentives for student behavior or to reward students?

- How important are the sales of SSBs for revenue (for food service, athletic department, administration)?

- How do you feel about SSBs being available at afterschool activities?

- Tell me about the availability of good-tasting, cold water throughout the day in your school.

In addition, information that might help with specific details of the intervention will be obtained through focus groups and interviews. For example, students and staff will be queried about the pros and cons of encouraging water dispensers at school, and students will be asked their opinions about potential logos and other promotional materials that the intervention team is considering.

From the student focus groups, the team hears that students know that water is healthier for them than SSB but see drinking SSB as the norm in their social groups. Although they are somewhat interested in the personal health aspects of consuming fewer SSBs and more water, what seems to energize them more are conversations about the impact of plastic bottles on the environment. This important insight provides the realization of a different "problem stream" that engages the students: the health of the planet rather than personal health. This insight will help in the development of activities for the classroom curriculum as well as messaging to be used with the social media component. From the school staff, the team learns that it is challenging to engage adolescents in traditional health education lessons; more experiential learning seems to work better. The team also hears that there has been some interest in reenergizing a school wellness council that has gone dormant. Some staff members believe that students and staff should be able to drink whatever they choose during the day, while others feel that school staff and school policy should facilitate and promote consumption of healthy beverages such as water.

The intervention team decides that a focus on the environmental aspects of choosing water over SSBs may garner more interest and support from both students and school staff as compared with a personal health approach. They decide to call the intervention "Healthy Teens, Healthy Planet" as a way to reframe the intent of the intervention. While approaching the issue from a different angle, the behaviors that will be addressed (reducing the intake of SSBs) and the determinants previously identified will remain the same. The team registers some resistance to policy and practice changes from some teachers, but they believe they have enough support to continue with that component.

Developing Strategies for the Curriculum Component
The team has decided that they will use a classroom curriculum with peer-led elements as the primary component to make a positive impact on determinants

from the individual-level environment. The intervention objectives to be addressed through the curriculum component are as follows:

- Enhance students' skills in being able to choose beverages without added sugar
- Increase students' awareness of price comparisons among SSBs, bottled water, and water dispensers in school
- Increase students' knowledge of what types of beverages include added sugar
- Increase students' knowledge about the healthfulness of water compared with SSBs

The intervention team focusing on the curriculum (including program staff, teachers, and curriculum specialists) brainstorm ways to achieve these objectives through a health curriculum for students in the seventh grade. Active engagement in learning is highly valued by the team; in addition, the team is well aware of the importance of social influence on eating behavior choices. The team also keys into the formative work reflecting a growing student interest in environmental concerns and the potential for student advocacy to reduce the impact of climate change. They decide to create a curriculum that includes peer-led, hands-on, group activities, adapting elements from the Teens Eating for Energy and Nutrition at School (TEENS) curriculum (Lytle et al., 2004), an evidence-based curriculum available from the National Cancer Institute's Evidence-Based Cancer Control Programs (http://ebccp.cancercontrol.cancer.gov).

To address the intervention objectives "enhance students' skills in being able to choose beverages without added sugar" and "increase students' knowledge of what types of beverages include added sugar," the team will adapt part of the seventh-grade TEENS curriculum that included class sessions involving hands-on, experiential learning stations led by peer leaders (Story, Lytle, et al., 2002). These learning stations included activities in which students considered the beverages that they typically consume during the day and introduced them to the amount of added sugars in beverages, including water, 100% fruit juice, milk, soft drinks, sports drinks, and other sugary drinks. To update this TEENS activity for the Healthy Teens, Healthy Planet intervention, the interventionists will add coffee drinks with added sugar and energy drinks as those beverages have become increasingly popular with adolescents in the past decade.

The team will create a new learning station activity as the intervention strategy to address the following intervention objectives: "increase students' awareness of price comparisons among SSBs, bottled water, and water dispensers in school" and "increase students' knowledge about the healthfulness of water compared with SSBs." This activity will involve calculating the cost per ounce of a variety of types and bottle sizes of SSBs and bottled water and comparing those prices with the one-time cost of buying a water bottle and using the water dispensers at school. In addition, the environmental cost of each of those beverage choices will be considered by examining estimates of the carbon footprint involved with producing SSBs in cans or plastic using estimates based on Footprint Expert 4.0 (Carbon Trust, 2012). To address the objective related to the healthfulness of water versus SSBs (both from a personal as well

TEENS EATING FOR ENERGY AND NUTRITION AT SCHOOL

TEENS was a multilevel, school-based intervention trial designed to evaluate the effectiveness of classroom, school-wide, and family programs to increase adolescent intake of fruits and vegetables and lower consumption of high-fat foods to reduce future risk of cancer (Lytle et al., 2004). The TEENS intervention included three components: (a) health curriculum developed for seventh- and eighth-grade classrooms, implemented by teachers and including a peer-led component; (b) family take-home packets that linked the TEENS curriculum with activities to be done with families and family incentives for making healthy behavioral choices; and (c) school-wide efforts to change foods and snacks available in snack lines, à la carte lines, and stores in the school and the use of a school nutrition advisory council to promote healthy, school-wide policy and practices. Details on the TEENS intervention, including the planning approach and the intervention strategies used, can be found in Lytle and Perry (2001).

The classroom component included 10 behaviorally based nutrition education lessons in the seventh and eighth grades. Both years of the TEENS curriculum included self-monitoring, goal setting, hands-on snack preparation, and skill development for choosing healthy foods and overcoming barriers to making healthful choices. Trained peer leaders were involved in seventh grade to help deliver segments of the classroom lessons. In eighth grade, behavior modification activities were included to help students see connections among cues, reinforcements, and their eating behaviors.

To complement classroom activities, families received three "Parent Packs" that contained activities and intervention-related messages. Each pack included a short family homework assignment; a newsletter with recipes and tip sheets on how to increase the availability of fruits, vegetables, and lower fat foods in the home; and 10 behavioral coupons with simple behavioral challenges such as "Serve a fruit and vegetable with dinner tonight." Families received a $10 gift certificate for returning 10 or more coupons.

Each TEENS intervention school had a School Nutrition Advisory Council (SNAC) made up of school administrators, staff, parents, students, and TEENS staff. The SNAC used a school-specific nutrition needs assessment (conducted by the TEENS staff) to make decisions about where to focus policy and practice changes. For example, SNAC activities included the development of policies and practices to limit the use of candy, sweets, and nonnutritious foods as rewards for student behavior or working with school staff to increase the availability of fruits, vegetables, and lower fat foods at school social and extramural events (Kubik et al., 2001).

as environmental standpoint), a series of short fact sheets will be created for the group to review; teams of students will compete in an interactive activity to determine which team knows the most facts. Water bottles will be given to the teams winning the most points. These intervention strategies employ a variety of the behavior change techniques (BCTs) described in Chapter 2. For example, BCTs from the domain "Shaping Knowledge" are used when students learn how to evaluate the amount of sugar available in commonly consumed SSBs. Likewise, BCTs from the domain "Associations" are used when students are taught how to be aware of and evaluate environmental cues prompting choosing water over SSB (Michie et al., 2013).

The final curricular activity will involve a project in which students estimate school-level consumption of drinks from bottled beverages (SSBs and bottled water) and create visuals to illustrate findings as a way to "increase students' knowledge about the healthfulness of water compared with SSBs" from a planetary perspective. Student pairs will interview at least five fellow students, teachers, and staff to get an estimate of how frequently they drink bottled beverages. Information collected by the class will be combined and based on the number of students, teachers, and staff in the school, an estimate of how many plastic beverage bottles the school contributes to landfills each year will be generated. These data will be used in a school-wide competition for the best graphic representation of the problem and will be part of the social media campaign. This change strategy involves elements of self-monitoring (Michie et al., 2013) and narrative engagement (Hecht & Krieger, 2006) and also uses a different problem in the problem stream (environmental consciousness as opposed to health concerns from SSBs) to help engage stakeholders (Kingdon, 2011).

Developing Strategies for the Social Marketing Campaign

The team developing the social marketing component will focus on the following intervention objectives:

- Decrease exposure to students and school staff drinking SSBs
- Increase exposure to students and staff choosing water as a beverage
- Increase the belief that many adolescents prefer water as a beverage
- Reinforce choosing water over SSBs

On the basis of information gleaned from the formative assessment, the social media component will present messages on the environmental impact of consuming beverages from plastic bottles and promote a normative switch from drinking SSBs and bottled water to using reusable water bottles and school water dispensers. The messages will include graphics depicting the number of plastic bottles in landfills and the effect on climate change; in addition, the positive impact of drinking fewer bottled beverages on climate change will be promoted. Students and teachers will be recruited to be involved in campaign messages to promote the switch to water at school and to serve as role models. A student contest to design the logo for a school water bottle will be conducted and water bottles distributed as incentives. The campaign will be shared through the school's Facebook and Instagram pages as well as through posters and intercom messages at school. The goal is to make drinking water from water dispensers the new normal.

For the social marketing campaign component, the intervention strategies draw on many of the change approaches discussed in Chapter 2 of this volume on the use of theories. BCTs (Michie et al., 2013) to be used will include "adding objects to the environment" from the Antecedents domain as water dispensers designed to fill water bottles are added throughout the school and "credible source" from the Comparison of Outcomes domain will be used as student and school staff role models speak out in favor of substituting water for SSBs. In addition, media messages can be developed to speak to students at different stages of change (i.e., those who are in the precontemplation stage and need to be convinced to switch versus those in the action phase that may need some tangible incentive to make the change; Prochaska et al., 2015). Diffusion of innovation (Rogers, 2003, Chapter 1) is particularly important for this component because the innovation (choosing water over SSBs; using water dispensers instead of buying bottled water or SSBs) will be introduced and reinforced through the social media campaign. In addition, the focus groups and interviews will help identify the innovators, or early adopters within the school, who can help lead the change effort. Importantly, using planetary health as the primary problem being solved reflects approaches suggested in the multiple-streams framework (Kingdon, 2011).

Developing Strategies for the Policy and Practice Component

The policy and practice component will work to address the following intervention objectives:

- Reduce the availability of SSBs on the school property
- Increase the accessibility of water on the school property
- Decrease the price of bottled water relative to the price of SSBs
- Make available and promote water dispensers throughout the school

Again, the team is able to draw on the TEENS program to identify intervention strategies to meet intervention objectives. The TEENS school policy component was developed using input from three sources: (a) an audit of foods and beverages available in vending and snack lines, (b) semistructured interviews with a school administrator to learn about school practices and procedures, and (c) a review of the school's written nutrition policy. In the TEENS study, data from these three sources were compiled into a needs assessment that provided a composite picture of the school's food environment. Each school's needs assessment was shared with school stakeholders, providing the starting point for discussion and decision-making (Kubik et al., 2001).

For the purpose of the Healthy Teens, Healthy Planet intervention, a process similar to what was done in TEENS will occur. Interviews and focus groups with school staff reveal that the school previously had a school wellness council but that it has not been active for a while. School administration and selected school staff are interested in revitalizing the council to support this component. The wellness council is reconvened to include a school administrator, two teachers, the school nurse, the food service manager, a parent and two students; a project staff will also attend council meetings to help facilitate the process.

The intervention team will obtain the school's written wellness and nutrition policy and conduct an audit of the physical environment including the following:

- number of varieties, bottle sizes of SSBs, and number of slots for each type of beverage available in vending, school stores, and on à la carte lines throughout the school (including soft drinks, sport drinks, energy drinks, sweetened teas, sweetened coffee beverages)

- price per serving of each SSB and any promotional information associated with the SSB

- locations where water is available throughout the school and how it is available (through bottled water or water dispensers)

- price per serving of bottled water and any promotional information associated with water

Data obtained from these semistructured interviews, the written wellness and nutrition policy, and information from the audit will be combined to create a needs assessment of the school food environment to be presented to the school's wellness council and used to help the school decide on its priorities for policy and practice initiatives.

The approaches used in this component reflect elements of intervention approaches suggested in the Multiple Streams Framework (Kingdon, 2011). The interviews with the school stakeholders are essential to understand other issues in the school's problem stream that might compete with or complement problems to be addressed through this intervention. Sharing the needs assessment with the school's wellness council is a way to explore potential policy options that might be helpful in positively influencing the school's beverage environment as well as a way to find program champions. Likewise, engaging a wide range of stakeholders as part of the school's wellness council helps engage the larger community (including parents and students) in the issue at hand, while the use of the school-specific nutrition needs assessment helps meet the community where they are and ensure the community can own whatever policy actions it decides to prioritize.

STEP 7: CREATE A LOGIC MODEL

The next step in the intervention design process is to create a logic model. Logic models are frequently used in public health as a way to plan, describe, manage, communicate, and evaluate a program or intervention (CDC, 2003) Logic models are visual representations of the theoretical and action components of the planned intervention and their expected outcomes. Logic models

INSIGHTS FOR INTERVENTIONISTS: CIRCLING BACK TO THE CONCEPTUAL MODEL

Once the team has a good idea of how each intervention objective will be met through the intervention components and strategies, it is good to plan a meeting to review the original conceptual model. The conceptual model provides the blueprint for the project, and before "construction" begins, it is important to verify that the intervention strategies planned will target the determinants identified in the Plan Phase. Sometimes drift occurs during the creative phase of the design process, leading to a mismatch between intervention strategies and the original intervention objectives. Sometimes this drift results when new stakeholders join the team or through a suggestion of some intervention idea that sounds particularly innovative or interesting. Confirming that the intervention strategies chosen will address the identified determinants is a good check on the process used to get the group to this point.

This review meeting is also a chance to see if something was missed or has changed in the community since the initial planning. Is the team satisfied that they have made the best decisions about the most potent and feasible approaches to use? Have there been any major changes in the community that would suggest that different determinants, intervention components or strategies should be considered? Big changes would have needed to occur to revisit existing plans, not just new hunches or new interests of a few stakeholders. If something has been missed or changed, it is better to make corrections to the intervention strategies now before additional resources are spent on intervention development.

can take several forms and serve different purposes, but in general, they are a schematic way to show (a) how determinants or factors are related to a health issue (this intervention design process refers to this schematic representation as a *conceptual model*), (b) the anticipated process of change (how the intervention strategies that are planned will affect change in the determinants), (c) components of the action plan (details on how the intervention strategies will be implemented), and (d) the expected outcomes (the health behavior to be changed by the intervention as specified in the conceptual model; Goodstadt, 2005). For the purpose of designing multilevel behavior change interventions, a logic model is used to add details to the intervention planning, including how many people are needed to execute each intervention strategy and what resources will be required at each phase in the project. The logic model is also used as a communication tool for other stakeholders, providing a visual representation of the planned program activities and their expected outcomes. The logic model is inextricably linked to the conceptual model and the intervention planning process that has already occurred.

Figure 4.1 shows a basic template for a logic model (CDC, 2003). The process side of the logic model describes the resources that will be needed for each of the intervention strategies that make up the intervention. The outcome side of

FIGURE 4.1. Sample Logic Model

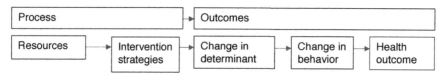

the model shows how each intervention strategy is expected to change the determinants of behavior, the behavior, and ultimately the health outcome of interest.

Example Logic Model: Healthy Teens, Healthy Planet

Figure 4.2 shows an example of the logic model for the Healthy Teens, Healthy Planet intervention. The logic model provides detail about the intervention activities, the materials needed, and the time required for each component's activities. For example, it specifies the number of peer-led classroom sessions involved in the curricular component as well as the time required to deliver, train, and prepare for the component and the materials that need to be prepared for each classroom session. Likewise, for the policy and practice component, details are included on all of the activities required, including collecting data for the needs assessment, convening and supporting the school wellness council, and the estimated time required for intervention staff to accomplish the tasks related to this component.

INSIGHTS FOR INTERVENTIONISTS: RESOURCES TO CONSIDER IN A LOGIC MODEL

The resources to consider in a logic model include personnel, products to be developed, and other tangible needs related to delivering the intervention. Identifying these resources is essential for estimating the costs of implementing each intervention strategy. A primary resource consideration is the personnel required to create and deliver the intervention strategy. This may include project staff, external businesses, consultants, and community stakeholders who have a role in creating or delivering the intervention. Estimates of how many staff members and what level of effort is required from them should be estimated for each intervention strategy. Likewise, material resources related to the implementation of each intervention strategy need to be considered, including producing or purchasing materials for the intervention; costs of creating websites, videos, or other platforms for delivering the intervention; and cost of incentives. Resource needs also include expenses related to training those delivering the intervention and expenses for creating and producing training manuals. In addition, some resources for communication are needed to keep participants and other stakeholders engaged and informed throughout the intervention.

FIGURE 4.2. Logic Model: Example From the Healthy Teens/Healthy Planet Intervention to Reduce the Intake of Sugar-Sweetened Beverages (SSBs)

Resources	Process	Outcome	
	Intervention Strategies	Determinant	Health Behavior
Classroom curriculum Session 1: Peer-led station activity-sugar content of beverages Session 2: Peer-led station activity-healthfulness of water and price comparisons Session 3: Group project-Estimating plastic bottle use by students, staff, and teachers	Create a 3-session, peer-led classroom curriculum using learning stations to achieve the following intervention objectives: • Increase students' confidence that they can make healthier beverage choices at school • Enhance students' skills in being able to choose beverages without added sugar	Perceived control	
Time required: Three classroom periods 45-minute training for the Peer Leaders 30-minute training for the teachers Approximately 40 hours of prep work for intervention staff	• Increase students' perceptions that healthy beverage choices are socially positive	Perceived barriers	
Materials to create: Peer Leader Guides/training materials Teacher Guide/training materials Student information sheets/worksheets	• Increase students' awareness of price comparisons between SSBs, bottled water, and water dispensers in school • Increase students' knowledge of what types of beverages include sugar • Increase students' knowledge about the healthfulness of water as compared to SSBs	Perceived knowledge	Adolescent consumption of sugar-sweetened beverages
Materials to assemble: _Session 1:_ • Assorted beverages with labels: water, 100% fruit juice, milk, soft drinks, sports drinks, energy drinks and sweetened coffee drinks • Props for the sugar-measuring activity • Worksheets for students			

(continues)

FIGURE 4.2. Logic Model: Example From the Healthy Teens/Healthy Planet Intervention to Reduce the Intake of Sugar-Sweetened Beverages (SSBs) (Continued)

Session 2: • Information on prices of a variety of beverages • Information on environmental costs of bottled SSBs and bottled water • Quiz sheets for competition • Water bottles for prizes *Session 3:* • Data collection sheets for each student pair • Worksheets for calculating beverage intake and estimate plastic bottle use • Guide for the data visualization competition			
Social Media campaign Media campaign to occur from September through November <u>Time required</u> Approximately 40 hours of preparation work <u>Materials to create</u>: Facebook and Instagram pages Posters to be displayed in the school	Create a social media campaign to achieve the following objectives: • Decrease exposure to students and staff drinking SSBs • Increase exposure to students and staff choosing water as a beverage • Increase beliefs that many adolescents prefer water as a beverage • Reinforce choosing water over SSBs	Observational learning/Role modeling Descriptive norm Social reinforcement	Adolescent consumption of sugar-sweetened beverages
Policy and Practices Activities will occur over the entire school year (August through May) <u>Activities required</u>: • Collect data on the school beverage environment for the school's nutrition needs assessment (intervention staff)	Work toward changes in policies and practices in the school. Use a needs assessment approach to describe beverages available in the school to the school wellness council and assist the school in establishing healthy beverage policies and practices to achieve the following objectives:	Availability of beverage choices as school	Adolescent consumption of sugar-sweetened beverages

- Create a needs assessment report to share with the school wellness council
- Assist in convening regular meetings (every other month) of the school wellness council
- Assist the school wellness council in identifying priorities for new policies and practices
- Support the school wellness council in implementing new policies and practices

Time required
School wellness council (approximately 6 meetings over the school year)
Intervention staff (approximately 15 hours/week over 9 months)
- Preparing needs assessment forms
- Collecting school-level data
- Preparing school needs assessment reports
- Presenting school needs assessment to school councils
- Attending regular meetings of the school wellness council
- Other supportive activities

- Work with school administration and staff to reduce the availability of SSB on school property
- With school administration and staff to increase the accessibility of water on school property
- Work with school administration to decrease the price of bottled water relative to the price of SSBs
- Work with school officials to promote students' use of water dispensers throughout the school

Relative price of beverages available at school (water vs. SSBs)

Note. Specific aim: The intervention will reduce students' daily mean consumption of sugar sweetened beverages by 50% of baseline consumption.

This is also a good time to create a timeline regarding how to prioritize activities. The team wants to enter the next phase of implementation reassured and confident that they have the staff, time, and resources needed to deliver the intervention strategies. Once the team is confident that the intervention is designed to be potent enough to change behavioral determinants identified during the Plan Phase and can be accomplished given the existing resources and timeline, it is time to share the plan with both the community and the evaluation team.

STEP 8: SHARE THE LOGIC MODEL WITH THE EVALUATION TEAM AND COMMUNITY STAKEHOLDERS

Convening a group of stakeholders to review the logic model provides an important opportunity to reengage the community in the project. Particularly for community stakeholders who have not been involved in the planning or creative process, presentation of the logic model helps to remind them of the set of determinants chosen during the Plan Phase to have a positive impact on the health behavior and provides a chance to review the intervention components and strategies. This process helps ensure that all stakeholders have a good understanding of what is going to happen, where it is going to happen, who will be involved, what resources are necessary, and the expected outcome of the effort. This process is an important step in engaging the community to think through any possible barriers to intervention implementation and to garner ideas about ways to use existing community assets to support intervention activities. Opportunities to build community capacity should be considered.

This is also the time to share final intervention plans with the evaluation team. The evaluation team will need to revisit the evaluation plans formulated during the Plan Phase and confirm how the dependent variable (the health behavior), the behavioral determinants, and the other modifying factors and covariates will be measured and the timeline for measurements. In addition, the logic model will also be useful in thinking through process evaluation needs as the inputs and resources needed for each intervention activity are highlighted. Process evaluation is discussed in the Implement Phase (discussed in Chapter 5), but, in brief, process evaluation is important in helping to document how the intervention was delivered and received. A carefully planned intervention that does not get delivered in the manner it was intended will have a diminished impact. Likewise, a carefully planned and well-delivered intervention will have limited impact if it is not received by its intended audience. To evaluate the effectiveness of an intervention, it must be delivered as planned (with fidelity), in the appropriate amount (dose delivered), and received by the intended audience (reach) at the intended dose (dose received). The evaluation team needs to be involved with identifying process measures because some evaluation resources will likely be needed in data collection, entry, and analysis.

At this point, it is important to confirm with the relevant stakeholders that there is general agreement about both the intervention and evaluation plans.

This general agreement can be confirmed through a memorandum of agreement (MOA), developed by the program planners and signed by the relevant parties. The MOA spells out the goals of the program, the general timeline of activities, the intervention components that will be used, the general evaluation plan, and a list of commitments that each stakeholder is making to the project. Although an MOA is not meant to be a legally binding document, it is extremely useful in confirming that all of the relevant stakeholders agree about the direction of the project. It is also a helpful document to have in case leadership of a major stakeholder changes midproject. Figure 4.3 shows a sample MOA that might apply to the Healthy Teens, Healthy Planet intervention.

This is also the time to make sure that the intervention manual of procedures that was introduced during the Plan Phase (Chapter 3) is updated. This update will include adding the logic model, a table showing intervention objectives, corresponding intervention strategies and intervention components, a projected timeline of intervention activities, a copy of all materials, and the protocol for how, and by whom the intervention is delivered.

SUMMARY OF THE CREATE PHASE

In the Create Phase, the team begins to design the intervention. Building on the previous work conducted during the Plan Phase, the team creates intervention objectives that clearly state how it will positively affect determinants of the behavior and decides on the components that will be used to meet the intervention objectives. With the help of creative people and with input from stakeholders, the team begins to develop the strategies that will make their intervention unique. This is the phase that moves from the conceptual to the tangible, and so a good dose of reality and practicality is needed; the team needs to create the most potent intervention possible with the resources and timeline available to them. As the intervention is being finalized, a logic model is created, building on the original conceptual model but adding important logistical and resource-specific details. At this point, circling back to community stakeholders is important to keep them informed and engaged and get them excited about the intervention. The evaluation team is getting all of the measurement tools ready before the intervention begins, so it is important to share the logic model with them to make sure that evaluation plans are thorough and complete. The team is now ready to move onto the Implement Phase, which involves developing process evaluation plans and finalizing intervention materials, training, and protocols.

FIGURE 4.3. Sample Memorandum of Understanding

Healthy Teens, Healthy Planet (HTHP) intervention: To reduce students' daily mean
consumption of sugar sweetened beverages

This Memorandum of Understanding (MOU) identifies elements of the partnership that will be
important in completing this research project.

ELEMENTS OF THE PARTNERSHIP:

I. The HTHP Program team agrees to:

1. Conduct all HTHP activities in a safe, professional, and sensitive manner. All HTHP staff
    will be clearly identified and follow all established school protocols in a manner agreed upon
    by school administration.

2. Provide development-training programs for all school and community personnel without cost
    to the school or community.

3. Provide all the equipment and materials needed to implement all aspects of the HTHP
    intervention.

4. Provide all needed resources to conduct the evaluation; be responsible for ensuring human
    subject protections are met and obtaining all required consent and assent.

5. Provide support for school and community members who are helping with the intervention
    and evaluation materials.

6. Appoint a staff member to serve as a member of the school wellness committee. This
    representative will attend collaborative partnership meetings to work on school-level policy
    and practice change.

II. The School Partner agrees to:

1. Support the logistics required for student recruitment and measurement activities.

2. Identify a school staff member who will serve as the liaison for coordinating HTHP
    measurement activities at their school. This school representative will assist the program staff
    in scheduling the recruitment and measurement activities at the school.

3. Identify a school staff member who is willing to serve as the intervention liaison and who
    will work with HTHP program staff to help coordinate intervention activities.

4. Provide physical space, when feasible, for HTHP activities occurring at the school, including
    intervention and evaluation activities.

5. Allow school staff involved with delivering elements of the intervention to attend trainings.

6. Allow HTHP social media messages to be distributed within the school.

7. Allow HTHP program staff to provide on-site assistance during the intervention to include
    feedback to teachers, technical support, model lesson segments, and answer questions.

The terms of this MOU will be _____ through _____.
                              (mo/day/yr)   *(mo/day/yr)*

This MOU shall be reviewed annually to ensure that it is fulfilling its purpose and to make any
necessary revisions.

On behalf of the school I represent, I am signing this MOU to be a partner in the WFW
intervention.

School partner representative/Date   Program representative/Date

_____   _____

5

The Implement Phase

The Implement Phase is the culmination of the Plan and Create Phases and provides the team their first glimpse of how the intervention may be received by its target audience. The first step in the Implement Phase is to develop process evaluation measures (Step 9). This chapter starts with an overview of the purpose of process evaluation and reviews its primary components (fidelity, reach, dose delivered, dose received, and context) and how each component is assessed. This section also includes a discussion of the special considerations for process evaluation for digital interventions. Examples of process evaluation from three multilevel intervention (MLI) trials are included, and this section ends with a discussion of how process evaluation may be used as part of quality control and in secondary and exploratory analysis. The chapter then covers Step 10—finalizing the intervention protocol, training, and materials—and addresses the importance of pilot testing an intervention, sources of information from the pilot, and how a team moves from the pilot study to an intervention. A review of developing needed materials, the importance of training, and updating the intervention manual of procedures is included under this step. The chapter ends with an example of how the Implement Phase would look for the hypothetical case study on developing a multilevel school-based intervention to reduce students' consumption of sugar-sweetened beverages (SSBs).

This phase includes the following two steps:

9. Develop process evaluation measures.
10. Finalize the intervention protocol, training, and materials.

https://doi.org/10.1037/0000292-006
Designing Interventions to Promote Community Health: A Multilevel, Stepwise Approach,
by L. A. Lytle

STEP 9: DEVELOP PROCESS EVALUATION MEASURES

The Purpose of Process Evaluation

Although outcome evaluation focuses on *if* an intervention worked to create change, process evaluation is the collection of data (both quantitative and qualitative) for the purpose of understanding *how* an intervention worked. Process evaluation allows us to determine the extent to which the intervention reached the target audience and how the audience responds to the intervention. Process evaluation provides information on how easy or difficult the intervention is to deliver and whether it is delivered as planned. It provides detail on the frequency and dose of the intervention as delivered by the intervention team and received by the target audience and can provide insight into how the dose received by the target audience is related to behavior change. It also helps us examine circumstances in the larger environment that may have had an impact on the intervention. Such information is critically important for explaining the results of interventions as well as providing insights for revisions, adaptations, and dissemination of the intervention. As public health interventions have become more complex, with intervention objectives targeting multiple levels of influence, with multiple audiences, and at multiple locations, the need to understand how an intervention is implemented, the extent to which it is implemented as planned, and how it is received by the target audience at each level has become increasingly important.

Unlike outcome evaluation, process evaluation data may be collected by those individuals conducting the intervention. For example, teachers delivering a classroom lesson may be asked to complete a process evaluation form. Process evaluation may also be collected by study staff through interviews, observations, or surveys. Unlike outcome evaluation, research or program staff may look at process data while the intervention is ongoing; if major problems with how the intervention is delivered or received are identified, midcourse corrections may be needed. More details on approaches for collecting process data are included later in this chapter. The textbook *Process Evaluation for Public Health Interventions and Research* (Steckler & Linnan, 2002) provides a thorough overview of process evaluation as well as detailed examples from community, worksite, school, and national and state process evaluation efforts and is a valuable resource for those new to process evaluation.

Primary Components of Process Evaluation

Many aspects of the intervention might be assessed as part of process evaluation, and decisions about the breadth and depth of process data to collect often come down to resources. At a minimum, process evaluation should include assessments of fidelity, reach, dose delivered, dose received, and context (Steckler & Linnan, 2002).

Fidelity

Fidelity evaluates the extent to which the intervention was implemented as planned. If an intervention is not delivered as planned, then neither success

QUESTIONS ANSWERED FROM EACH PROCESS EVALUATION COMPONENT

- **Fidelity:** To what extent was the intervention implemented as planned?
- **Reach:** To what extent did the intervention reach the intended audience?
- **Dose delivered:** To what extent was the full dose of the intervention delivered to the target audience?
- **Dose received:** What level of dose did each participant receive?
- **Context:** What other factors in the larger environment influenced the outcomes of the study?

nor failure of behavior change can be attributed to the intervention, and little will be learned about the intervention to inform future efforts. Lack of fidelity represents a Type III error, or error due to an intervention not being properly implemented (Basch et al., 1985).

Fidelity reflects the clarity of the intervention protocol, how well interventionists are trained to deliver the intervention protocol, and the feasibility of delivering the protocol in a real-world setting. For an intervention to be implemented with fidelity requires that those delivering the intervention have an excellent understanding of what, how, when, and how frequently intervention strategies are to be delivered. This information is included in the intervention manual of procedures (IMOP) and is communicated through intervention training. Any confusion or ambiguity in the written procedures or in training threatens fidelity. Those delivering the intervention need to be trained in the specifics of each intervention strategy and how they are to be delivered. Although the IMOP provides a written way to present that material, training is required to make sure that the information is understood and the importance of delivering the intervention as planned is reinforced. Fidelity is also threatened when the implementation of the protocol runs into significant barriers in the field. For example, an intervention trying to limit workers' consumption of SSBs in a worksite by changing the availability of products in vending machines may run into problems during implementation if the contract with the vending machine company limits their ability to specify product placement. Likewise, fidelity will be threatened if an intervention relies on clinic staff to deliver a health message, but the staff finds it nearly impossible to deliver messages because of time constraints. The use of a pilot test is extremely important in identifying unexpected barriers before the full implementation of the intervention or program and is discussed later in this chapter.

Ensuring that the intervention is being delivered with fidelity is an important and ongoing responsibility of the intervention team. Anything that threatens implementation as planned should be identified early and corrections or adaptations made quickly.

Reach

Reach is the proportion of the intended audience that participates in the intervention and provides insight into its relevance to the audience targeted and

INSIGHTS FOR INTERVENTIONISTS: HOW TO RESPOND WHEN PROCESS DATA SUGGEST A PROBLEM

When process data suggest that the intervention has not been delivered with **fidelity** or problems with **dose delivered** are seen, it is important to examine the following:

- **The intervention protocol:** Is it clearly written? Is it complete?

- **The intervention training:** Was everyone who had some responsibility for delivering any aspect of the intervention trained? Were new staff trained as they joined the project team?

- **Oversight of the intervention delivery during the intervention trial:** Was there a process for reviewing how the intervention was being implemented during the trial and making midcourse corrections?

When process data suggest that **reach or dose received** is an issue, it is important to examine the following:

- **The relevance and importance of the intervention:** How relevant is the intervention or program for the intended audience? What are the competing priorities for the target audience that may limit interest and participation?

- **Logistical challenges limiting participation:** Were there significant logistical challenges, such as when, where, and how the program was offered, that influenced participation? Did issues with childcare or transportation keep the target audience from participating?

- **Costs of participation:** Was participation impacted by the cost of participating, including money, time, or hassle?

- **Appropriateness of the intervention for the community:** Did the target audience feel comfortable with how the program was promoted and conducted? Were those delivering the intervention respectful of the community's culture? Were the intervention activities and materials appropriate for the target audience?

When process data suggest that context is an issue, it is important to consider the following:

- **The interpretation of findings:** To what extent are the results of the study influenced by external events or potential confounders that have little to do with actual intervention activities?

its generalizability to specific audiences. Reach includes an assessment of the success of recruitment strategies to attract the target audience as well as participation of the target audience in intervention activities. As an example, if a clinic-based intervention identifies low-income women as its target audience for prenatal classes, assessing reach will involve examining the proportion of low-income women who sign up for the classes relative to other income groups who enroll (recruitment success) as well as assessing the income characteristics of those attending the classes. Similarly, for a school-based intervention targeting foods available in the school cafeteria, reach may examine the types of schools that are more likely to agree to participate in the intervention (e.g., rural vs. urban schools or private vs. public schools) and the school characteristics represented by the food service workers who attend training.

Dose Delivered

Dose delivered refers to the amount of the intended intervention that program participants receive. The intervention's Create Phase includes careful consideration of the intervention dose required for behavior change. Dose is reflected in the number of intervention components and strategies planned to meet intervention objectives and the amount of time dedicated to intervention activities.

Dose delivered reflects an aspect of fidelity but includes more qualitative aspects of the intervention delivery. For example, an intervention relying on sending text messages as behavioral cues and reinforcements may specify in the protocol that four text messages per week will be sent; however, due to staffing issues, only two text messages per week are sent. Alternatively, a group training session is scheduled to last 45 minutes, but some of the sessions are shortened to 25 minutes due to challenges in scheduling a room for the sessions. In these examples, it is apparent that aspects of the intervention strategies may be delivered with fidelity, but the interventionists are unable to deliver the full dose of the intervention.

Dose Received

Dose received refers to the extent to which participants actively engage with the intervention. Interventions are designed to deliver each participant a "dose" of the intervention that is expected to result in behavior change. If the individual does not fully engage with the intervention, then behavior change is threatened. Dose received may reflect an individual's motivation to participate or external barriers that prevent them from fully participating in the intervention. Although dose delivered reflects how interventionists deliver the intervention, dose received reflects how participants respond to it. For example, a web-based intervention to encourage young adults to be more physically active includes an opportunity for goal setting and tracking minutes of activity per day. Assessing the number of goals set and the behaviors monitored by each participant through website data analytics represents a measure of dose received or active engagement with the intervention strategies. Likewise, a pregnant woman may sign up for three prenatal group sessions that focus on helping her control her Type 2 diabetes. The number of sessions that she actually attends represents the dose she received.

The concepts of reach and dose received are similar in that both consider who "shows up" for intervention activities. They are different in that reach refers to the proportion of the intended audience that is involved with intervention activities while dose received refers to the proportion of the intervention that is received by an individual participant. Using the example of group sessions designed for pregnant women with Type 2 diabetes, reach attempts to measure the proportion of women enrolled in the program who show up for one or more sessions and answers such questions as the following: Were first-time mothers more likely to attend at least two sessions compared with mothers with at least one child at home? Were mothers on medical assistance more likely to attend sessions compared with mothers with private insurance? In contrast, dose received examines an individual's degree of engagement with the intervention and related factors. Dose received answers such questions as the following: Did mothers who attended at least two of the three sessions have lower blood sugar levels at the end of the intervention as compared with mothers attending only one session? Was the number of sessions attended related to women's perceptions of social support?

Context

Context (also referred to as secular trends) reflects things happening in the larger environment that may directly or indirectly affect the implementation of the intervention and interpretations of the study's findings. Context includes occurrences in the larger social, political, or economic environment that are beyond the control of the intervention or program staff. Context is especially important for understanding the results of an intervention trial when both the intervention and control conditions are influenced by changes in the larger environment.

Context is one of the more challenging process measures to plan for because it involves anticipating events that might occur in the larger environment with a potential to influence the study's results. This type of process data may pick up secular trends that will influence behavior in the intervention and control conditions, mitigating the ability to detect differences attributable to the intervention. As an example, a worksite wellness intervention may have a goal of increasing employee consumption of fruits and vegetables through a variety of worksite programs and incentives. The team plans to randomize worksites and compare employee consumption patterns between worksites randomized to receive the intervention and worksites randomized to the control condition. Several things could happen after randomization that could affect the study's ability to see differences between the treatment conditions, including a state-wide media campaign encouraging everyone to eat more fruits and vegetables, a change in the company's vending contract that results in more fresh fruits and vegetables in all worksites, or an increase in the presence of farmers' markets near the worksites. Such changes in the larger environment might influence consumption patterns of employees in both the intervention and control conditions, making it difficult to see differences between the groups or attribute change to the intervention.

Process Evaluation Measurement and Methods

Table 5.1 provides a summary of measurement considerations for each of the five main process evaluation components, including the treatment groups involved in the data collection, typical type of data collection method, and the frequency of data collection.

Assessing Fidelity and Dose Delivered

Fidelity and dose delivered are assessed using the same tools and may include logs, recordings of intervention sessions, and checklists. Logs are used to provide

TABLE 5.1. Process Evaluation Components

Component: question answered	Treatment condition	Data collection methods	Timing frequency

Fidelity: To what extent was the intervention implemented as planned?	I	• Logs
		• Session recordings/ transcripts
		• Checklists
		  – Evaluator observation
		  – Interventionist self-report
			• At each intervention session or at a subsample of sessions

Reach: Did the intervention reach the intended audience?	I	• Attendance logs • Surveys or interviews assessing relevant participant characteristics	• When recruited/ enrolled in study • At each intervention session

Dose delivered: To what extent was the full dose of the intervention delivered to the target audience?	I	• Logs
		• Session recordings/ transcripts
		• Checklists
		  – Evaluator observation
		  – Interventionist self-report
			• At each intervention session or at a subsample of sessions

Dose received: What level of dose did each participant receive?	I	• Attendance logs • Other metrics assessing engagement • Surveys	• At each intervention session • Throughout the intervention • Midcourse/ post-intervention
Context: What other factors in the larger environment might have impacted the implementation of the intervention and the outcome of the study?	I and C	• Surveys • Interviews • Archival data	• End of the study at a minimum • Pre, post, and midcourse is optimal

Note. C = control; I = intervention.

basic information on the intervention session, including when it began and ended, where it was held, and the name of the interventionist leading the session. Logs should be completed for every session by the interventionist leading the session or by an evaluation staff member observing the session. Logs also provide information on dose delivered because they are used to document occurrences that might have interrupted a session, prevented it from being delivered as planned, or prevented a "full dose" of the intervention. (As an example, in schools, fire drills are often the culprit when intervention activities are disrupted.) Occasionally, group- or individual-level counseling or educational sessions are audio recorded to evaluate fidelity and dose delivered. Project staff review session transcripts to document the content as delivered and to confirm that the major points of the intervention were delivered as planned. Data collectors reviewing the transcripts are encouraged to make notes to highlight any quality control issues that need to be addressed. Using a checklist to document fidelity or dose delivered involves creating a data collection form that lists the core elements of the intervention activity or session. The data collector is asked to record whether the element was covered (yes–no) and the fidelity with which the core element was covered (high, moderate, or low). Either an evaluation staff member or the interventionist delivering the session completes the checklist.

Cost and resources often dictate the mode of data collection as well as who collects the data. Having evaluation staff collect the data improves the validity of the data but adds additional cost and logistical challenges. When it is not economically or logistically feasible for evaluation staff to attend or listen to all intervention sessions in all locations, a plan to collect a representative sample of the intervention sessions is required. A less expensive way to collect information on fidelity and dose delivered is to have the interventionist delivering the intervention complete a checklist at the end of each session. Although this approach allows all of the intervention sessions to be evaluated, it has the disadvantage of potential bias because most interventionists intend to deliver all of the intervention with high fidelity and want the audience to be fully engaged.

Assessing Reach

Reach is measured by collecting data on the characteristics of those participating in the intervention. Data on reach are collected through attendance logs, surveys, interviews, or other data collection methods that capture the characteristics of those who agreed to participate as well as those who showed up for each intervention session or activity. Reach is examined at the aggregate level (i.e., the proportion of the sample from a specific subgroup), not the individual level (i.e., the number of times that an individual attends an intervention session, representing dose received). It is difficult to assess reach for interventions that target unspecified audiences where individuals are not enrolled in the study, such as social media or promotional campaigns. For example, estimating the reach of a promotional campaign to encourage workers to use the stairs is challenging because it is impossible to know the characteristics of those employees who noticed the signage near the stairs or read the flyers and promotional materials about the benefits of using the stairs. We can describe the characteristics of workers, but we cannot describe the characteristics of those workers who actively engaged with the intervention. Some policy interventions have the advantage of having 100% reach. As an example, policies that eliminate smoking in public places may have close to 100% reach, depending on the degree to which the policy is enforced.

Assessing Dose Received

Dose received can be assessed using attendance logs, other metrics that indicate engagement with the intervention activities, and surveys. Attendance logs that include the names of the participants present at each session are essential for establishing dose received. At the end of the planned intervention sessions, the proportion of sessions attended by each participant can be used as one estimate of dose received. Dose received can also be estimated using specific metrics of engagement. For example, in a study using goal setting and behavioral monitoring as an intervention strategy, counting the number of times goals are set and behaviors are recorded can serve as a measure of engagement. Likewise, in a study using community engagement strategies to impact policies and practices, the number of times that a stakeholder representative attends planning meetings represents dose received. Unfortunately, there is no easy way to estimate cognitive engagement with intervention content; participants may be physically present but inattentive and not actually receive the intervention's full dose.

If an intervention is delivered through social media (e.g., an online campaign to reduce vaping among young adults) or depends on health communications delivered to a large audience (e.g., a newsletter mailed to older adults in a retirement community), assessing the dose received by the target audience is challenging because it is difficult to assess the number of times and the amount of time individuals spend with the intervention material. Surveying intended recipients is one of the few ways to evaluate whether intervention strategies are received. Survey respondents may be asked to identify content, including media messages, slogans, or program titles that were used in the intervention. Confederate messages, slogans, and program titles are included along with the intervention's actual messages, and participants' ability to identify the intervention messages is used as an estimate of dose received.

Assessing Context

Of the five process evaluation components, only data regarding context are collected in both control and intervention conditions because external environmental influences may affect both conditions. The three collection methods typically used to collect contextual data are surveys, interviews, and archival data. Survey questions are commonly used if the data are to be collected before, during, and after the intervention; interviews may be used for less frequent data collection or with fewer anticipated respondents. Planning survey questions to assess context is difficult because doing so requires anticipating situations or occurrences that could conceivably happen during the intervention period. Open-ended interviews with key stakeholders allow a fuller exploration of environmental changes that may have influenced the behavior of interest. Surveys or interviews are conducted with administrative or organizational leads in the intervention and control conditions by evaluation staff.

Using archival data available for the communities involved in the intervention may also contribute to an understanding of contextual influences. Archival data may include any type of public record that describes some aspect of a community environment. For example, for an intervention designed to increase levels of activity in a community, data from a city's Parks and Recreation Department on the number and size of parks and recreational centers in an area could be examined to see if new opportunities to be active occurred during the intervention period. Likewise, for an intervention designed to increase community members' intake of fruits and vegetables, commercial or public health data on the number of full-service grocery stores, convenience stores, and farmers' markets in the community may be useful sources of information related to potential environmental impacts on consumption patterns. At a minimum, contextual data should be collected at the end of the intervention period; additional data collection periods—for example, baseline and mid-intervention—are optimal. The review of archival data is done by evaluation staff.

Special Considerations for Evaluating Digital Interventions

There are some unique considerations for collecting process evaluation for digital interventions. Fidelity and dose delivered are assessed in similar ways as face-to-face sessions using interventionists or evaluation staff to confirm the protocol was delivered as planned. For digital interventions, process evaluation measuring fidelity and dose delivered might include the number of text messages or emails sent by the interventionists or the number and frequency of phone calls made to participants. For digital interventions that recruit and enroll participants, reach is relatively easy to assess, but for interventions conducted on the internet without limiting access to participants, collecting such data is difficult because the denominator of those exposed to the intervention is unknown.

Assessing dose received is a particular challenge with digital interventions. If a web-based intervention asks recipients to post comments on message boards or enter self-monitoring behavioral data, reliable information on dose received can be collected. The number of comments posted and the number of self-monitoring data entries can be counted and used as an estimate of relative engagement. Likewise, a qualitative content analysis can be conducted with the comments posted to help understand how members of the target audience interacted with the intervention and content. It is difficult to know how and how long people engage with digitally presented information, even using web-based analytic tools. The length of time the website is open may reflect the amount of time the individual was on the website reading material or may simply reflect that the website was opened but the participant moved onto other activities without logging out. Conversely, the individual may have opened the website, printed the content, and closed the website. Logins to an intervention website or "hits" to specific pages provide some data regarding dose received, but it is difficult to evaluate how engaged participants were with the content. For interventions relying on text messages and email to provide information or prompts, it is often impossible to know whether a text message or an email message was opened or, if opened, actually read. Methods for quantifying engagement with digital interventions are currently being developed (Miller et al., 2019).

Other Considerations for Choosing Process Evaluation Measures

In addition to these five process measures, many other pieces of information might help explain how the intervention worked. For example, Baranowski and Stables (2000) suggested that there are 11 components of process evaluation: recruitment, maintenance, resources, barriers, initial use, continued use and contamination, in addition to context, reach, implementation (fidelity), and exposure (dose received). Each process evaluation component to be measured requires resources and imposes some cost or burden for intervention and evaluation staff, and potentially, the target audience. The intervention and evaluation team must work together to determine which components are most essential for understanding how the intervention worked and for considering the needs, wants, and concerns of relevant stakeholders (Steckler & Linnan, 2002).

For intervention components and strategies that have been used before, fewer process evaluation measures might be needed. But for components and strategies that have not been widely used, more process evaluation might be required to better understand how well the protocol and training worked, identify any issues regarding the feasibility of delivering the intervention, and identify how the target audience responded to the components and strategies. Finally, a mix of quantitative and qualitative data should be collected for process data. Quantifiable measures are important because of their ability to be translated into variables that can be considered analytically. However, qualitative data using focus groups and interviews from stakeholders provide critical information on how the content and delivery of the intervention could be improved to better meet community needs. These stakeholders include both the audience that received the intervention and those delivering it.

Finally, it is essential that process evaluation is planned for each intervention component reflecting all of the environmental levels targeted in the MLI. Because there are so many moving parts in an MLI, understanding how each part is delivered and received is critical. Process evaluation can be used to explore the relationships and synergy between levels and may be useful for generating new hypotheses about how the levels interact. The next section provides examples of process evaluation methods used in MLIs.

Examples of Process Evaluation in Three Multilevel Interventions

Three interventions serve as examples of the use of process evaluation in MLIs: Teens Eating for Energy and Nutrition at School (TEENS), Choosing Healthy Options in College Environments and Settings (CHOICES), and the Trial of Activity in Adolescent Girls (TAAG).

TEENS

The TEENS intervention was described in the Create Phase (see Chapter 4). Briefly, TEENS was a school-based intervention trial designed to evaluate the effectiveness of an MLI to increase adolescents' intake of fruits, vegetables, and lower fat foods. Sixteen schools were randomized to either a control or intervention condition, and a cohort of 3,878 seventh- and eighth graders was recruited to participate in the study. The TEENS intervention lasted 2 years and targeted all three environment levels (individual, social, and physical) through three components: classroom curriculum in seventh grade and eighth grade, a family component in both seventh and eighth grades, and a school-wide policy and practice component. The classroom curriculum was taught by schoolteachers, mostly through the family and consumer science classes, and each year included 10 behavior-based nutrition education lessons; some sessions in the seventh-grade curriculum were peer led. The family component was delivered in conjunction with the classroom activities. Parents received "Parent Packs" that contained a short homework assignment to be done with parents, a newsletter with recipes and tip sheets, and 10 behavioral coupons that could be redeemed for a gift certificate. The school-wide policy and practice component was organized around each school's School Nutrition Advisory Committee (SNAC) made up of school administrative staff, the school nurse, food service staff, teachers, students, and one TEENS staff member. On the basis of each school's needs assessment, each SNAC worked on policy and practice approaches to positively influence students' exposure to fruits, vegetables, and lower fat foods while at school (Lytle et al., 2004, 2006; Lytle & Perry, 2001).

Table 5.2 shows the process measures collected for each of the three components of the intervention (Story et al., 2002). Process measures related to the classroom curriculum included assessing teacher and peer leader training and, in both cases, included log sheets to document that training occurred, training attendance, and a short survey at the end of training to obtain participants' level of engagement with the training and general insights. Reach, dose delivered, engagement, and general insights were collected through these methods. The fidelity with which the classroom curriculum was delivered was assessed by observations of the class sessions by study evaluation staff and by reviewing the self-assessment checklists teachers completed at the end of each session. Figure 5.1 shows an example of the TEENS classroom session checklist. Feedback was obtained 2 weeks after the end of the curriculum from teachers, students, and peer leaders either through a structured interview (teachers) or a brief survey (students and peer leaders). This data collection method was used to obtain an assessment of engagement and general impressions of the curriculum and included questions, such as: "What lessons did you think were the most/least effective?" (teachers), "How helpful were the peer leaders?" (students) and "My friends thought it was cool that I was a peer leader" (peer leader). Process evaluation for the TEENS family component was limited to assessing reach and dose delivered by counting the number of Parent Packs returned without being delivered to parents and a count of the number of behavior coupons returned from each family. The school policy and practice

TABLE 5.2. Teens Eating for Energy and Nutrition at School (TEENS) Process Evaluation Measures

Intervention component	Aspects	Methods	Frequency	Process components
Classroom curriculum	Teacher training	• Log sheet (attendance, length) • Teacher survey (feedback on training)	• At each training event	• Reach, dose delivered • Engagement, general insights
	Peer leader training	• Log sheet (attendance, length) • Peer leader survey (feedback on training)	• At each training event	• Reach, dose delivered • Engagement, general insights
	Delivery of classroom lessons	• Classroom observation by evaluation staff • Checklist completed by teachers	• Four of 10 sessions each year (randomly chosen) • After each session	• Fidelity, dose delivered
	Teacher feedback	• Structured interview	• 2 weeks after the completion of the curriculum	• Engagement, general insights
	Student feedback	• Survey	• 2 weeks after the completion of the curriculum	• Engagement, general insights
	Peer leader feedback	• Survey	• 2 weeks after the completion of the curriculum	• Engagement, general insights
Family component	Parent packs	• Number of parent packs returned/ number of parent packs mailed	• After each mailing (three times/year)	• Reach
	Behavioral coupons	• Number of possible coupons returned/ received (30 coupons/ year)	• End of each year	• Reach • Dose received

(continues)

TABLE 5.2. Teens Eating for Energy and Nutrition at School (TEENS) Process Evaluation Measures (*Continued*)

Intervention component	Aspects	Methods	Frequency	Process components
School policy and practice	School Nutrition Advisory Council (SNAC) meetings	• Number of SNAC meetings • Log sheet (attendance, length)	• Throughout the year • Each meeting	• Reach, dose delivered • Reach, dose delivered
	Teacher engagement with food-related policy and practice	• Teacher survey	• End of each school year	• Reach, dose received, general insights
Intervention as a whole	Principal feedback	• Structured interview	• End of each year	• Context

component was assessed by tracking the number of SNAC meetings held at each school and attendance at each of those meetings throughout the year. At the end of each school year, teachers were asked to complete a survey that tapped their engagement with school food-related policy and practice. A structured interview was also held with each principal in all 16 schools to get their general impressions of the intervention as a whole and included questions to assess contextual factors that might have influenced the study. For example, principals were asked, "In the past year, did your school have any special activities related to health promotion topics such as 'National Nutrition Month' or a '5-a-Day and fruits and vegetables program'?"

CHOICES

The CHOICES intervention was part of the Early Adult Reduction of weight through LifestYle intervention (EARLY) trials (Lytle, Svetkey, et al., 2014) and was a 24-month weight-gain-prevention intervention for young adults (Lytle, Moe, et al., 2014; Lytle et al., 2017). CHOICES enrolled 441 participants from three 2-year community colleges in Minnesota. These students were randomized to a control or intervention condition after baseline data were collected. The CHOICES intervention worked at the levels of the individual and social environment and included two components: an academic course and a social network website. Participants randomized to the intervention condition enrolled in a 1-credit, semester-long academic course (created and paid for by the study) that was offered in three formats: face-to-face on site at their community college, online, and through a hybrid model. Students chose their preferred course delivery option. The hybrid model included all lessons online, but students were expected to be on campus for four in-person sessions: a cooking class, a physical training class, a yoga class, and a stress-reduction class. CHOICES intervention staff were responsible for delivering all of the classes, but a faculty member from each college served as the instructor of record. The course was offered for two semesters in each school. In addition to the required course, participants in the intervention condition were encouraged to participate in a social network and

FIGURE 5.1. Sample TEENS Classroom Observation Checklist

Please complete this form for each session that you teach. The questions are repeated three times to allow you to use the same sheet if you teach multiple classes.

SESSION ONE: INTERVIEWS

TEACHER:

Class hour: |__|

Grade level |__|__|
Minutes per class period: |__|__|
Number of students in the class: |__|__|
Number of Peer Leaders present: |__|__|
Who taught the class? *(Check one)*

1 ☐ Teacher
2 ☐ Substitute Teacher
3 ☐ Student Teacher
4 ☐ Other: _____

1. **Session One included the following activities. Which did you teach?**

	Yes	Partly	No
a. Introduction - Peer Leaders	1 ☐	2 ☐	3 ☐
b. TEENS Interview Video	1 ☐	2 ☐	3 ☐
c. Sampling Snacks	1 ☐	2 ☐	3 ☐
d. Assignment	1 ☐	2 ☐	3 ☐

2. **Did you like teaching this session?** 1 ☐ 2 ☐ 3 ☐

3. **Did the students enjoy this session?** 1 ☐ 2 ☐ 3 ☐

4. **How well did the Peer Leaders do the following tasks?**

	Very Well	Okay	Did Not Do
a. Introduce TEENS	1 ☐	2 ☐	3 ☐
b. Lead the video activity	1 ☐	2 ☐	3 ☐
c. Keep their group on task	1 ☐	2 ☐	3 ☐

5. **Check any activities that were particularly successful.**

a. 1 ☐ Introduction - Peer Leaders
b. 1 ☐ TEENS Interview Video
c. 1 ☐ Sampling Snacks
d. 1 ☐ Assignment
e. 1 ☐ Rating Snacks

Class hour: |__|

Grade level |__|__|
Minutes per class period: |__|__|
Number of students in the class: |__|__|
Number of Peer Leaders present: |__|__|
Who taught the class? *(Check one)*

1 ☐ Teacher
2 ☐ Substitute Teacher
3 ☐ Student Teacher
4 ☐ Other: _____

	Yes	Partly	No
a.	1 ☐	2 ☐	3 ☐
b.	1 ☐	2 ☐	3 ☐
c.	1 ☐	2 ☐	3 ☐
d.	1 ☐	2 ☐	3 ☐

1 ☐ 2 ☐ 3 ☐

1 ☐ 2 ☐ 3 ☐

	Very Well	Okay	Did Not Do
a.	1 ☐	2 ☐	3 ☐
b.	1 ☐	2 ☐	3 ☐
c.	1 ☐	2 ☐	3 ☐

a. 1 ☐ Introduction - Peer Leaders
b. 1 ☐ TEENS Interview Video
c. 1 ☐ Sampling Snacks
d. 1 ☐ Assignment
e. 1 ☐ Rating Snacks

Class hour: |__|

Grade level |__|__|
Minutes per class period: |__|__|
Number of students in the class: |__|__|
Number of Peer Leaders present: |__|__|
Who taught the class? *(Check one)*

1 ☐ Teacher
2 ☐ Substitute Teacher
3 ☐ Student Teacher
4 ☐ Other: _____

	Yes	Partly	No
a.	1 ☐	2 ☐	3 ☐
b.	1 ☐	2 ☐	3 ☐
c.	1 ☐	2 ☐	3 ☐
d.	1 ☐	2 ☐	3 ☐

1 ☐ 2 ☐ 3 ☐

1 ☐ 2 ☐ 3 ☐

	Very Well	Okay	Did Not Do
a.	1 ☐	2 ☐	3 ☐
b.	1 ☐	2 ☐	3 ☐
c.	1 ☐	2 ☐	3 ☐

a. 1 ☐ Introduction - Peer Leaders
b. 1 ☐ TEENS Interview Video
c. 1 ☐ Sampling Snacks
d. 1 ☐ Assignment
e. 1 ☐ Rating Snacks

Note. Subscript numbers by response options are used for data coding.

support website that was designed specifically for the CHOICES study. Students were introduced to the website during their course and encouraged to continue using it during the 2-year intervention period. The website was open only to intervention participants and a limited number of their invited guests. The website was designed to reinforce, inform, and encourage exchange and support between participants. Participants were encouraged to log their weight regularly and to set goals for weight-related behaviors (e.g., eating fast food, fruits, and vegetables; eating breakfast; eating mindfully; screen time, sleep, and stress management) and to support each other in their behavioral goals. The website included articles, recipes, quizzes, and numerous ways to accumulate points for prizes (Lytle, Moe, et al., 2014; Lytle et al., 2017).

Table 5.3 summarizes the process evaluation for CHOICES. The process evaluation for the academic course included attendance at the face-to-face classes and the required in-person sessions for the hybrid class option (Laska et al., 2016). Logins were counted for each participant in both the online and hybrid options. These measures allowed us to assess reach and dose delivered. Completed assignments were counted as a measure of dose received. Attendance and assignments were counted using the Desire2Learn course management system (https://www.d2l.com/) that was in place in the three community colleges. To assess the fidelity with which the classes were delivered and the dose delivered, CHOICES instructors completed a checklist at the end of each face-to-face or hybrid in-person session. To assess dose received and engagement, students completed a survey where they provided an estimate of how many hours per week they were interacting with course materials and the degree to which they completed each lesson. Students in all three course delivery options completed this survey, but the frequency with which they completed them differed. As part of the process data for the academic course and to assess engagement with the intervention, students were asked at the end of the semester about their satisfaction with the course. For example, students were asked whether they found the course material interesting and whether they had been able to understand the course content. In addition, students who were not engaged with the course were invited to participate in a brief interview at the end of the course to learn about their barriers to participation. The instructors of record from each school were interviewed each semester to obtain their impressions of the course and how students responded to it. For example, the faculty were asked to comment on which aspects may have facilitated or posed barriers to student involvement with the course.

Process data related to the social networking website focused on assessing reach and dose received and were collected using web-based analytics. Data collected included engagement with the behavioral goal and self-monitoring aspects of the website, as well as participation in social network opportunities on the website. The number of logins, the number of times participants posted their weight, the number of behavioral goals set, and self-monitoring activities were all counted. Likewise, the number of times a participant posted a reinforcement or support of another student's goals or behavior, posted information for the network, or responded to another's post was tracked as an indication of reach

TABLE 5.3. Choosing Healthy Options in College Environments and Settings (CHOICES) Process Evaluation Measures

Intervention component	Aspects	Methods	Frequency	Process components
Academic course: college course (1 credit; sleep, eat, exercise and stress): offered face-to-face; hybrid model; online	Attendance	• Face-to-face class: Desire2Learn learning management system, log sheets (attendance) • Attendance at in-person sessions (hybrid) • Logins to lessons (hybrid and online)	• Each of 16 classes • After each of four in-person sessions • Each login	• Reach, dose delivered
	Assignment completion	• Face-to-face class: Desire2Learn learning management system (grades entered) • Online documentation	• After each assignment • At end of four content areas	• Dose received, reach
	Delivery of classroom lessons	• Checklist completed by instructors (face-to-face)	• After each session	• Fidelity, dose delivered
	Student engagement with lessons: hours interacting with course materials; degree to which lessons were completed	• Student survey	• Twice within the semester (face-to-face) • After each of four content areas (hybrid, online)	• Dose received, engagement
	Satisfaction with the course	• Student Survey • Interview with students that did not fully participate	• End of the semester	• Engagement, general insights
	Instructor of record impressions	• Interview with instructor of record	• Once each semester	• General insights/ impressions

(continues)

TABLE 5.3. Choosing Healthy Options in College Environments and Settings (CHOICES) Process Evaluation Measures (*Continued*)

Intervention component	Aspects	Methods	Frequency	Process components
Social network website	Behavioral goal setting and self-monitoring	• Number of logins • Number of times weight was posted • Number of behavioral goals set • Number of times self-monitoring a behavior	• Throughout the intervention	• Reach, dose received
	Participation in social network activities	• Number of times posted a reinforcement to someone's goals or self-monitoring • Number of times posted information • Number of times responded to others' posts	• Throughout the intervention	• Dose received
	Overall engagement in website	• Points awarded for participating in website activities	• Throughout the intervention	• Reach, dose received

and dose received. To estimate overall engagement with the website, students could earn points for tracking a behavior, posting a comment, updating their status, or setting a goal. Points could be redeemed for a gift certificate or other item of their choice related to healthy living and provided another estimate of reach and dose received (Laska et al., 2016).

TAAG

TAAG was a multicentered group- or cluster-randomized intervention trial testing a school and community-based intervention to prevent the decline of physical activity in middle school girls. The TAAG trial was conducted at six university-based field sites representing different geographic locations across the country. Six schools at each of the field sites were randomized to a control or intervention condition after the completion of baseline data. The TAAG intervention targeted the individual, social, and physical environments and consisted of four components: TAAG Physical Education (PE), TAAG Health Education, TAAG Programs for Physical Activity, and TAAG Promotions. TAAG PE involved training each school's PE teachers to deliver a curriculum that promoted activity for all students during PE time. Each teacher received training, a teacher's guidebook, task cards, and an activity box. TAAG Health Education included six classroom lessons for seventh- and eighth graders that promoted the development of behavioral skills related to physical activity and included an activity challenge with behavior goal setting and self-monitoring as homework. Schools could decide whether TAAG Health Education was taught in a regular classroom setting or as part of PE. TAAG Programs for Physical Activity involved a collaboration between the community and the school, looking for ways to provide appealing, active programming for girls through after school and community-based opportunities. This component involved collaborating with local fitness studios, the local YWCA, and activity clubs to link girls with existing activities or to create new activities specifically geared toward adolescent girls. Finally, TAAG Promotions involved a social marketing campaign in each of the TAAG intervention schools that included posters and messaging in school and at special events to promote girls activity. Many of the campaign messages focused on social norms and supporting an active lifestyle for girls (Elder et al., 2007; Stevens et al., 2005; Webber et al., 2008; Young et al., 2006).

Table 5.4 shows a summary of the process evaluation for TAAG. The process evaluation measures for TAAG PE and Health Education included attendance logs at each teacher training to assess reach and dose delivered. In addition, TAAG evaluation staff observed training to document the fidelity with which training was delivered by TAAG intervention staff. Process data assessing the fidelity and dose delivered for class sessions were obtained through staff observations at selected classes. The sampling scheme created ensured that each teacher was observed the same number of times during different class periods and on different days of the week. Observations occurred approximately six times in each class per semester and documented key elements, such as teachers providing choices for activity options during class or using strategies to limit class management time. In addition, PE teachers completed a survey at the end of each school year to report on their use of the teacher guidebooks, task cards, and activity boxes. For TAAG Health Education, logs of the proportion of girls in each class completing activity challenges were maintained to represent dose received and reach. Finally, from this component, each teacher using TAAG PE or Health Education was interviewed at the end of the school year to assess their general level of engagement in the curriculum and to obtain other insights (Young et al., 2008).

Process evaluation for the Programs for Physical Activity included structured interviews with principals to learn about their links to community agencies offering activity opportunities for girls as well as surveys with sponsors of physical activity in the community to learn about any activity programming being planned. These interviews and surveys were done with both control and intervention schools in the Spring semester as a way to assess context. Reach and dose delivered were assessed through attendance logs kept at TAAG-related programming throughout the 2-year intervention. The process evaluation to assess dose received and reach for TAAG Promotions included a student survey completed by girls in both the control and intervention conditions to see if girls

TABLE 5.4. Trial of Activity in Adolescent Girls (TAAG) Process Evaluation Measures

Intervention component	Aspects	Methods	Frequency	Process components
TAAG Physical Education (PE) and Health Education	Teacher training	• Logs (attendance, length) • Observations	• Each training session	• Reach, dose delivered • Fidelity
	Delivery of classroom lessons	• Staff observations • Teacher survey	• Approximately six times per semester/ school • End of the school year	• Fidelity, dose delivered
	Health education activity challenges	• Logs of girls completing challenges	• End of the semester	• Dose received, reach
	Teachers' perceptions	• Structured interviews with teachers	• End of the school year	• Engagement, general insights
Programs for Physical Activity	Links between schools and community	• Structured interviews with principals	• Spring semester	• Context
	Availability of school and community activity programs	• Surveys with sponsors of physical activity programs	• Spring semester	• Context
	Girls' participation in TAAG programs	• Logs (description of program, length, attendance)	• Throughout the intervention	• Reach, dose delivered
TAAG Promotions	Exposure to the promotional messages	• Student survey	• Spring semester	• Dose received, reach
	Participation in special events (passport challenge in seventh grade; pedometer challenge in eighth grade)	• Logs	• For each event	• Dose received, reach

exposed to TAAG would be able to recognize the slogans and messages used in promotional efforts. For example, actual messages included in the promotional activities included "Real girls, real activities, real fun" and "Get active, stay active"; confederate messages included "Play sport: it's good for you'" and "Eat right, stay strong, live longer." Reach and dose received were also assessed through logs and counts of participation in student-centered challenges designed to encourage activity (Young et al., 2008).

The Use of Process Data for Quality Control, Secondary Outcomes, and Exploratory Analyses

Unlike outcome evaluation, process evaluation can be reviewed during the trial as part of quality control activities. Process data collected during the trial may reveal issues that threaten the integrity of the trial, instigating midcourse corrections. Although major changes to the intervention should not occur midstream (the determinants chosen for change, the intervention objectives and strategies designed, and the components for delivering the intervention should not change once the intervention has started), other issues around delivery may be identified through the process evaluation and addressed to enhance the implementation of the intervention. As an example, in TAAG, a 2-day, off-site, centralized training of PE teachers for each of the six TAAG sites and 18 schools was planned. All of the PE teachers involved with delivering the intervention were brought together at a central location at their respective university sites and trained by TAAG intervention staff. The training included discussion about the objectives and rationale for TAAG as well as introducing, demonstrating, and practicing recommended elements of a TAAG PE class, including class management activities to minimize inactive time, ways to provide students choice in activities, and how to organize activities by group sizes to promote activity by all students (Young et al., 2008). Shortly after the intervention began, we realized that many teachers, across all of the TAAG field sites, were having difficulty implementing lessons as planned. Rather than let the teachers continue to struggle for the remainder of the school year, we supplemented the original training with additional onsite training in each school. TAAG study interventionists scheduled regular visits with PE teachers to help them run the lessons until they became comfortable with the new format of classes. TAAG interventionists continued to offer support to the teachers throughout the intervention, as was originally planned.

Variables representing process data may be used to evaluate hypotheses for secondary outcomes. For example, hypotheses related to intervention dose are frequently included as secondary outcomes. It is intuitive to expect that those who were more engaged in and received a higher dose of an intervention would have greater levels of behavior change compared with those receiving a smaller dose. A stratified analysis in which dose received is categorized into levels of high, medium, and low can be used to examine how different levels of dose are related to behavior change, including the control group as the primary comparison group. Likewise, a study may include a secondary outcome that tests differential response to an intervention by reach. For example, a worksite intervention to increase physical activity levels of workers may hypothesize that the intervention will be more effective in females compared with males or in clerical staff compared with management. Process data collecting the characteristics of those recruited for and engaged in the intervention activities will allow those types of secondary outcomes to be evaluated.

Most components of process data (with the exception of context) are available only for those units randomized to the intervention condition, meaning that a true control group is not available for statistical comparison of effectiveness. Still, process data can be used in exploratory analysis and may be useful in examining trends and generating hypotheses to be tested in fully powered and randomized trials. As an example, the TEENS study evaluated the effectiveness of a multilevel school-based intervention to positively influence fruit, vegetable, and lower fat food intake in seventh- and eighth graders. After baseline data collection, schools were randomized to a control or intervention condition, and students within schools provided the behavioral data on which TEENs was evaluated. TEENS was fully powered to examine the impact of the entire intervention on differences at the school level, but within the intervention schools, all students did not receive the same intervention dose. All students in the intervention schools were exposed to a school-wide environment that reflected changes to food-related policy and practice, but because of students' class schedules and course requirements, not all students in each intervention school received the TEENS curriculum. In addition, a small group of students in each intervention school were chosen as peer leaders in seventh grade, receiving additional training and engaging at a different level in curricular activities. Therefore, students within each intervention school received a different dose of the intervention. It would seem plausible that those students who were peer leaders, received the TEENS curriculum, and were exposed to school environmental changes might experience a larger behavior change compared with students receiving a smaller dose.

Using process data identifying the aspects of the intervention delivered to each participant, we were able to examine the influence of four different doses of intervention received on fruit, vegetable, and fat intake between baseline and the end of the first year of the intervention. Those included (a) no intervention received by students in schools randomized to the control group; (b) students exposed only to school-level environmental policy and practice changes; (c) students receiving the TEENS curriculum and the school-level environmental changes; and (d) students who were peer leaders, received the TEENS curriculum, and were exposed to school-level environmental changes (Birnbaum et al., 2002). As expected, patterns suggesting a dose response were observed, with peer leaders reporting the largest increases in fruit, vegetable, and lower fat food consumption. Students exposed to classroom plus school-level environmental changes also showed significant change in positive eating behaviors, whereas students exposed only to school-level environment interventions showed trends toward choosing lower fat foods and declining fruit intake but no change in vegetable intake. Control student's food choices remained stable over the year.

TEENS was not designed to be able to answer questions regarding which components were most effective in fostering behavior change. Evaluating the effectiveness of individual levels of an intervention, specific intervention components, or interactions between levels and components would require schools to be randomized into each component (Cleary et al., 2012; Murray et al., 2010). Such a study design would have required recruiting many more schools into the study and many more resources. Short of that type of study design, these process data help examine the relationship between the dose received and behavioral outcomes and are useful in suggesting questions to be explored further in fully powered trials. For example, because peer leaders experienced the greatest behavior change, is there some way to involve more students in leading aspects of a classroom curriculum? Because exposure to just the changes in the school environment resulted in the least amount of behavior change, what other strategies must accompany environmental changes to help energize change (Birnbaum et al., 2002)?

STEP 10: FINALIZE THE INTERVENTION PROTOCOL, TRAINING, AND MATERIALS

The last step in the Implement Phase involves finalizing the intervention protocol, training, and materials. Typically, and ideally, a pilot test of the intervention or program is conducted before the intervention, and its related materials are finalized.

The Importance of a Pilot Test

A pilot test is essential when implementing a new intervention for the first time and provides a practice run of the intervention before it is evaluated for effectiveness in a fully powered intervention trial (Whitehead et al., 2014). Pilots allow the intervention team to observe how the intervention is delivered and received. Process evaluation collected during the pilot can help identify strategies that are difficult to deliver because of their complexity or strategies that are not feasible because of limitations of the setting or time constraints. Likewise, the pilot can help reveal an intervention strategy that does not engage the audience. Although the pilot attempts to deliver as many aspects of the intervention protocol as possible, some components may be difficult to pilot. For example, an intervention component that involves changing an institution's policy and practice may be difficult to pilot because of the time required to engage the stakeholders in the issue, work through barriers to change, and obtain organizational commitment to change. On the other hand, it is relatively easy to pilot a curriculum, a new approach for group counseling, or a social marketing strategy.

The pilot also provides the opportunity to test the data collection protocol for outcome and process data to be used during the main trial. As data are collected in the pilot, better estimates of the time required to collect the data, issues with the data collection forms, burden to respondents, questions that arise from those completing the measures, and other challenges to data collection can be revealed and used to modify the protocol for the main trial. The pilot is an important opportunity to train interventionists and data collectors and to see where the protocol may be unclear or particularly challenging to execute and where training needs to be modified. The pilot also provides an opportunity to gain insight into the protocol for recruiting and retaining participants. Issues that arise can be brought back to stakeholders for advice and suggestions on appropriate changes for the main trial.

A pilot is conducted with a small sample that closely matches the target audience intended for the full intervention trial or program. For example, if the intervention is to be conducted across community centers in an urban area, the pilot should be conducted in one or two of the centers. Alternatively, if the intervention involves group classes, the pilot should occur with a small number of groups using the planned recruitment strategy within the targeted audience. Those involved in the pilot (e.g., individuals, community centers, schools, worksites) should be excluded from participating in the main trial because of their exposure to the intervention; they would come with prior intervention experience and "contaminate" the study design. Typically, the same stakeholders who will deliver the intervention in the main trial conduct the pilot intervention; if worksite team leaders will deliver the intervention in the main trial, they should be trained to deliver it in the pilot. Likewise, data collection activities should be conducted by the same group that will collect data in the main trial. A pilot trial may be conducted with both an intervention and a control condition, but the goal of the pilot is not to evaluate effectiveness; the sample size of a pilot trial will be insufficient for that purpose. Still, the inclusion of a control group allows investigators to examine potential issues around recruitment and retention, pilot any intervention to be offered in the control condition, and look for trends in behavior change (Whitehead et al., 2014).

Sources of Information From the Pilot Test

Lessons are learned through the pilot from four sources: (a) firsthand observation of intervention and data collection activities, (b) process evaluation data, (c) additional qualitative information, and (d) examination of trends in change in the determinants and outcome.

It is important that the intervention developers are committed to full involvement in the pilot, including firsthand observation of each element of the intervention. This is not the time to rely on staff to run the intervention and report back; this is the opportunity to observe how the interventionists deliver the intervention and how the target audience responds. Intervention developers need to be able to see participants' level of engagement and notice when interventionists struggle with delivering content. In addition, those responsible for evaluation efforts need to be on-site when data are collected to observe how the process for data collection works in the field. If there are issues with training or feasibility, the pilot phase is the time to identify those problems; identifying data collection problems once baseline data collection has started is stressful and requires a quick and immediate response.

Process data should also be collected during the pilot as a way to see how the intervention seems to work. Process data showing issues with lack of fidelity of implementation suggest there are aspects of the intervention delivery that are cumbersome to deliver in the field or issues with training. Likewise, process evaluation data measuring reach and dose delivered may reveal an issue with attracting the target audience or implementing the full intervention protocol as intended. Process measures assessing dose received may identify a need to find additional or different ways to engage the target audience in intervention activities.

The pilot is an excellent opportunity to collect qualitative information on how a variety of stakeholders respond to the intervention. As interventionists and data collectors engage in pilot activities, their feedback on training, the questions raised regarding implementation, and their insights into how well the protocol was delivered in the field are important to receive and document. In addition, conducting focus groups or interviews with the target audience engaged in the pilot intervention can help refine intervention strategies, materials, and messages and even provide insights into preferred incentives, logos, and other marketing materials. Even informal conversations with those delivering the intervention and members of the target audience can provide invaluable insight into improvements to be made for the main trial.

Finally, although the pilot will typically not include a sample that is large or representative enough to allow an evaluation of its impact on the determinants or outcomes to be evaluated, pilot data are often used to examine trends in impact. Pilot data that show change in the right direction for determinants and the behavioral outcome suggest that the intervention has the potential to be effective in a fully powered trial. This evidence may be helpful in obtaining additional funding for a larger trial or in garnering continued community support for ongoing intervention work. If no trend toward positive impact is seen in the pilot, before conducting the larger trial, the team should consider the fidelity with which the pilot was delivered; the content of the intervention, including the dose, intervention components and strategies; logistical or feasibility challenges encountered; and the sensitivity of measurement tools.

How to Move From a Pilot Study to an Intervention Trial

The intervention team should meet regularly during the pilot phase of the study to discuss what is going well and what modifications are needed before the main intervention trial is launched. Changes should not reverse the important work done in the planning phase; the determinants targeted and intervention objectives should remain constant. In most cases, the intervention components will also remain constant from the pilot to the main trial because components are chosen based on the intervention objectives to be met and with input from the stakeholders. Pilot testing may reveal that intervention strategies are not

SOURCES OF INFORMATION FROM A PILOT TEST

- **Field observations of intervention and data collection activities:** Lead developers of the intervention and evaluation efforts observe the implementation of the intervention and data collection activities.

- **Process evaluation data:** Process evaluation conducted during the pilot provides important insights into potential issues to be addressed.

- **Qualitative data:** Planning interviews or focus groups with those delivering and receiving the intervention, data collectors, and other key stakeholders will provide important information on any necessary revisions to the protocol.

- **Examining trends in change in determinants and outcomes:** Results from the pilot suggesting that trends for change are in the right direction build confidence in the approach.

working and new strategies to address intervention objectives may need to be developed. If time allows, pilot testing new strategies is recommended. The time between the pilot and the main trial depends on the complexity of the intervention. Even a simple intervention likely requires at least 3 months between the end of the pilot and the beginning of the intervention trial to modify protocol, materials, and training.

INSIGHTS FOR INTERVENTIONISTS: FUNDING FOR PILOT STUDIES

Funds to pilot an intervention may be found through existing funding mechanisms available to organizations or through small grants. The justification for a pilot is that the money requested is to support pilot work to be used to develop a proposal for a fully powered effectiveness study. The National Institutes of Health (NIH) uses the R34 Planning Grant Program to fund pilot intervention work. This mechanism allows 3 years of funding for a maximum of $250,000 per year and a maximum of $450,000 in direct costs. The R34 specifically identifies "pilot studies or collection of feasibility data for subsequent research projects" (NIH, n.d., see Introduction) as the type of research supported under the mechanism. Five-year grant awards from the NIH such as an R01 might allow for a short pilot, time to revise the intervention based on the pilot, and a fully powered intervention trial. NIH funding for fully powered intervention trials that include a pilot in the timeline often require that some feasibility work reflecting proof of concept has been completed. Pilot work is a good investment of time and money for both funders and those funded.

Types of Intervention Material to Be Developed

Finalizing the needed materials is an important step toward implementing the intervention. These include materials individual participants will receive, materials that will be used to engage the community or organization in intervention activities, and materials needed for training. Materials needed for individual participants will include all content designed to instigate and support behavior change, including the lessons, worksheets, videos, and support materials that are used for curricula; the website and all content to be presented on the website; podcasts to be used; and text, email, and phone messages to be sent as part of a digital intervention. In addition, many interventions create materials to support retention of study participants—for example, postcards with birthday greetings, small prizes for when goals are met, or text or email messages to remind participants to log into the website. Materials are needed to communicate organizational and logistical information to the community and other stakeholders, including consent and assent forms, contact information, and details about how, when, and where participants are involved in intervention activities. Materials also need to be finalized for the interventionists; these include session objectives to be covered, sample scripts for virtual or group counseling sessions, and all training materials. Templates for all of these materials can be developed before the intervention begins, with details added as the intervention unfolds.

Some thought also needs to be given to the types of materials needed for interventions that focus on organizational or policy change. These types of intervention often are more process than content oriented, and while the intervention objectives are clear, development of the intervention is more fluid, making it difficult to design the relevant materials before the intervention activities begin. However, often some approaches and related materials to guide the process can be developed ahead of time. As an example, CounterTools is a nonprofit organization with the goal of advancing public health by enacting and enforcing policy, systems, and environmental interventions that promote health equity across communities (https://countertools.org/). In particular, it works with communities to reduce the impact of unhealthy substances such as tobacco, alcohol, and unhealthy food in the retail environment. CounterTools's process for change begins by documenting the local problem through a needs assessment with community partners to better understand the retail environment. A data visualization process transforms those data into infographics, maps, and other charts and visual aids that helps a community "see" the issue in their community more clearly. CounterTools also generates reports that analyze the current environment and provides insights into potential policy approaches. Although every community's project is different, policy work is facilitated by the creation of a system and software that drives data visualization and reports (Myers et al., 2019).

Once an intervention begins, the entire intervention team becomes busy; therefore, anticipating all the materials that will need to be written and produced before the intervention starts creates an efficiency the entire team will appreciate. Once the intervention begins, needs for additional supportive intervention materials may be realized and will have to be created. Likewise, sometimes small changes need to be made to intervention materials as the intervention training or implementation rolls out. Additions and small edits are to be expected. Interventionists should avoid the need to produce major intervention content and material once the intervention has begun. All materials produced should include a completely digitized version to facilitate the documentation and dissemination of the intervention and related materials.

The Importance of Training

Training those who will be delivering the intervention is an essential part of the Implement Phase. The approach to designing MLIs to promote population heath used in this book engages community in all aspects of intervention planning, creating, implementing, and evaluating and uses all of those phases as opportunities to build community capacity. Therefore, in many cases, those delivering the intervention will be community members who have little training in health or how to foster health behavior change in others (e.g., teachers, worksite leaders, youth development professionals, spiritual and religious leaders). Training provides the basics they need to know about the health behavior, the related health outcome, and how to help create change. Even when trained health professionals, including nurses, counselors, community health workers, worksite wellness coordinators, or graduate students in health-related programs, will be delivering the intervention, training on how to deliver the specific protocol is required. Training helps the interventionists understand the importance of adhering to the intervention protocol, how to respond appropriately to questions and issues that arise, and to grasp the specifics of delivering each intervention component.

Training begins with developing training manuals and sessions specific to each component and strategy. The intervention team must train all individuals who will be delivering the intervention; a centralized session in which all are trained at the same time is optimal. Using a "trainer of the trainers" approach is not usually as effective because pieces of the protocol are often missed, or instructions misinterpreted as the training responsibilities move further from the intervention team. Training the entire intervention team at the same time permits questions and issues that arise to be immediately clarified for all involved. Even if different interventionists deliver various components of the intervention, having a centralized training session in which some of the entire intervention team spends time together is helpful to show interventionists how the components are integrated. Understanding the big picture may lead to a greater understanding of and appreciation for what the intervention is to achieve and the importance of adhering to the protocol.

Training should be engaging, interactive, and encourage questions and discussion. It should involve experiential learning in which attendees see pieces of the intervention modeled and have the opportunity to practice delivering various elements. A training limited to a presentation of the material or an overview of the intervention manual will quickly lose attendees' interest and threaten the likelihood that the intervention will be delivered as planned. Community-based trainees are often shy about expressing what they do not understand about the health behavior and are reticent to ask questions. Interventionists should come up with creative ways to engage trainees and thus provide good learning opportunities. For example, in CATCH (see Chapter 1), we trained classroom teachers to deliver lessons to third-, fourth-, and fifth graders on eating a healthy diet and the importance of physical activity. We began their training with a short and fun true–false quiz that elicited common misconceptions or confusing points about healthy eating and activity. The teachers were surprised at how many questions they missed, and their results instigated a lively discussion that clarified many points of confusion. That activity early in the training also led the way to more open discussions, questions, and clarifications as the training day continued.

Training should occur as close as possible to the beginning of the intervention so that attendees begin using the information they have learned immediately. Depending on the complexity and length of the intervention, additional training or individual trainings may be warranted. For long interventions, booster trainings may need to be planned not only to support the original interventionists trained but also to provide training for new interventionists.

Updating the Intervention Manual of Procedures

During the pilot and active phases of the intervention, the IMOP is a crucial source of information. It is used to document the decisions made throughout the intervention design process and to orient new project team members and stakeholders who become involved with the project during the design process. The IMOP represents the criterion measure, or gold standard, against which the process data collected during the intervention trial or program will be compared. The IMOP describes the intended dose and delivery of the intervention as well as the materials or intervention content to be delivered to the audience at specified times.

The details that are added to the IMOP during the Implement Phase include the following (see Exhibit 3.2 for a list of all of the information to be included in the IMOP):

- For each environmental level, include
    1. descriptions of how each intervention component will be implemented, including timing, dose, who delivers the intervention strategy, and materials needed
    2. details on what occurs at each session or each contact point with participants
    3. copies of all materials produced, such as written materials, text messages, internet-based materials (e.g., website content, posts, content for social media, scripts for interventionists)
    4. other level-specific protocol and correspondence

- Intervention standardization, including the following:
  1. training needs, training protocol, and related training materials
  2. the process for intervention team communication (e.g., plans for providing rapid feedback on the intervention, fidelity checks, retraining needs)
- Plans for collecting process data and the related process forms
- Any changes in protocol as the intervention proceeds

The IMOP describes how each component is designed to work and includes details on what will occur at each contact point for an individual or group. For example, if an intervention component includes group counseling sessions, the specific goals, objectives, and activities of each session should be detailed in this manual. In addition, all materials to be used in each session should be included. For example, if text messages will be sent as prompts and reinforcements for behavior, the protocol regarding when they are sent, sample content of the messages, and guidelines for follow-up should be described. All materials produced for each component are documented in the IMOP; these may include correspondence to participants, worksheets for classes, website screenshots, content for social media posts, background materials for developing policy briefs, and data shared with policy makers.

The IMOP also includes information and materials related to standardizing the delivery of the intervention, such as details on how interventionists are trained, the timing and frequency of training, certification and retraining, and all related training materials. The manual also details the process of quality assurance for the intervention delivery, including how to provide rapid feedback to interventionists, how adaptations to the intervention occur, and how to determine retraining needs. Likewise, the manual covers details on the process evaluation, including how and by whom process data will be collected and all data collection forms. The IMOP is meant to be a living document that reflects how the intervention was originally designed to be delivered and any minor modifications made to it during implementation.

When the intervention is completed, the IMOP is important source material for professional reports or published articles that result from the work. In addition, the IMOP is essential for sharing intervention details with other groups interested in replicating or adapting the intervention, providing detail far beyond what is typically available in summary reports about the effectiveness of the intervention or in published articles. It is increasingly recognized that crucial information is lost when published papers and summary reports are relied on to describe an intervention (de Bruin et al., 2021; Hoffmann et al., 2013; Lorencatto et al., 2013; Wadden et al., 2006). Requests for intervention materials from the authors too often result in unanswered requests or, at best, piecemeal provision of selected materials. Although there is a move to provide in-depth intervention materials through electronic supplements and providing open-source materials, this practice is not yet widespread. These limitations make it nearly impossible to understand how the intervention worked (or didn't work), determine the most essential elements to include in replications, and

TIDᵢₑR: A METHOD FOR IMPROVING THE REPORTING OF INTERVENTIONS

The TIDieR (Template for Intervention Description and Replication) is an extension of the work done as part of the Consolidated Standards of Reporting Trials (CONSORT) and the Standard Protocol Items: Recommendations for Intervention Trials (SPIRIT; Chan et al., 2013; Schulz et al., 2010). It represents an effort to improve the description of intervention trials. The TIDieR checklist (Hoffmann et al., 2014) encourages those reporting the results of an intervention trial to include details such as the following:

- name of the intervention
- rationale, theory, or goal of the essential elements
- all materials used, including those given to participants, training materials, and information on how the information can be accessed
- procedures, activities, and processes used to instigate change
- the category of intervention provider (i.e., nurse, community health worker, teacher)
- mode of delivery (i.e., face-to-face or group; individual vs. group session)
- where the intervention occurred
- dose, duration, intensity, and timing of intervention activities

provide guidance on how to adapt the intervention. Therefore, a commitment to create an IMOP that is designed to be shared is one of the most important things a team can do to help advance practice and science. Intervention details that the intervention team develops and revises throughout the design process should be easily accessible in the manual. Providing intervention details enhances the ability to replicate or build on intervention research approaches and findings. Without such documentation, researchers and practitioners have little chance of learning from experience. The field is responding to this need for more detailed information on interventions by calling for systems that promote more transparency (Hoffmann et al., 2014).

Example of Finalizing Intervention Protocols: Healthy Teens, Healthy Planet

In the previous descriptions of the Plan and Create Phases, I used an example of designing a multilevel school-based intervention to reduce student consumption of SSBs, "Healthy Teens, Healthy Planet." In this section, I use this example to illustrate pieces of the Implement Phase, specifically choosing process evaluation, what a pilot might look like, and material and training needs.

A description of the Healthy Teens, Healthy Planet, intervention is included in the Create Phase (see Chapter 4, this volume); in brief, the intervention includes three components: a three-session classroom curriculum with peer leaders, a school-wide social marketing campaign, and activities to change school-wide policy and practice. For the curriculum, peer leaders will lead two station activities that provide experiential, hands-on activities related to identifying and choosing beverages that are lower in sugar and increasing awareness of the healthfulness of water and the environmental implications of beverages sold in plastic bottles. Classroom teachers will oversee the station activities and will also lead the third session, which involves having students survey peers and school staff about their typical beverage choices. Through this activity, the class will estimate the grams of sugar consumed by students and staff and the number of plastic bottles that these consumption patterns contribute to landfills. The curriculum will be offered throughout the year as schedules permit in appropriate classes.

The social media campaign will occur during the fall semester and include media messages and images designed to increase social norms around choosing water over SSBs as a beverage option and using reusable water bottles and school-wide water-filling stations instead of plastic bottles. The campaign will occur via the schools' Facebook and Instagram pages as well as through posters in the school and via intercom announcements.

The third component will take place over the entire school year and involve helping school stakeholders make changes in school-wide policies and practices to reduce student and staff exposure to SSBs and to encourage their consumption of water using reusable water bottles. A school nutritional needs assessment will be conducted at the beginning of the year to identify potential areas for change, and a school advisory council will be assembled to lead the change.

Process Evaluation Plans

Table 5.5 shows the process evaluation plan for the intervention. For the curricular component, process data will be collected on attendance at training for both the peer leaders and teachers to assess reach and dose delivered. In addition, teachers and peer leaders will complete a brief survey at the end of training to assess how well they understood the protocol, their confidence in being able to deliver the curriculum, and their general level of engagement with the activities. Because of limited resources, the fidelity with which the peer leaders and the teachers deliver the three sessions will be assessed using a checklist completed by the classroom teacher at the end of each session. At the end of each curricular module in a class, all students will be asked to complete a brief survey to assess their level of engagement with curricular activities (dose received) and to collect insights on how the curriculum was received by students. At the end of the curriculum module, teachers and peer leaders will be invited to participate in a short, structured interview to obtain their feedback on the delivery of the curriculum, students' reactions to it, and recommendations for revisions.

Process evaluation for the social media campaign will involve counting "likes" and posts to the schools' Facebook and Instagram pages as well as a brief student survey at the end of fall semester to assess students' ability to recognize the major media messages used during the campaign. Process evaluation for

TABLE 5.5. Sample Process Evaluation for the Healthy Teens/Healthy Planet Intervention to Reduce Intake of Sugar-Sweetened Beverages (SSB)

Intervention component	Aspects	Methods	Frequency	Process components
Classroom curriculum	Peer-leader training	• Log sheet (attendance, length) • Peer leader survey (feedback on training)	• At training • Following training	• Reach, dose delivered • Engagement, general insights
	Teacher training	• Log sheet (attendance, length) • Teacher survey (feedback on training)	• At training • Following training	• Reach, dose delivered • Engagement, general insights
	Delivery of classroom lessons	• Checklists completed by teachers	• After each session	• Fidelity, dose delivered
	Student feedback	• Brief survey completed by all students completing the curriculum	• End of the curriculum	• Dose received, general insights
	Peer-leader feedback	• Structured interview	• End of curriculum	• Engagement, general insights
	Teacher feedback	• Structured interview	• End of curriculum	• Engagement, general insights
Social media campaign	Facebook/ Instagram	• Number of likes/ comments	• End of the first semester	• Dose received, general insights
	Overall campaign	• Student survey: recognition of media messages	• End of the first semester	• Dose received
Policies and practices	School wellness council	• Log sheet (attendance, length) • Number of council meetings	• Each meeting • Throughout the year	• Reach, dose delivered • Reach, dose delivered
	School staff recognition of beverage policies	• Teacher survey	• At baseline and end of year	• Dose received
Intervention as a whole	Principal feedback	• Structured interview	• Baseline and end of year	• Context, general insights
	Food service manager feedback	• Structured interview	• Baseline and end of year	• Context, general insights

the policies and practices component includes logs and attendance at each school wellness council meeting and a count of the number of meetings held throughout the school year. Because the intent of the policy and practice component is to have an effect on the larger school environment, a baseline teacher survey will be planned, and at the end of the school year, teachers' recognition of intervention activities will be assessed as a measure of dose received. Finally, to collect information on contextual occurrences that might have influenced the intervention and to gain general insights into the intervention as a whole, structured interviews will be conducted with each school principal and food service manager for the control and intervention schools at baseline and at the end of the school year.

Planning the Pilot Intervention

For this example, assume that the intervention is to be evaluated in a large suburban school district that includes 20 middle schools. Before a full evaluation of the intervention is conducted, the appropriate stakeholders will choose a school from the district to pilot the intervention. Good candidates for the pilot school would have very engaged teachers and administrators, be proximal to the university or health department conducting the intervention research, and have district leaders who support the project. The pilot will focus on implementing the classroom curriculum and the social marketing campaign. All aspects of the classroom curriculum will be piloted, including teacher and peer leader training, the two peer-led sessions, and the group activity. All aspects of the social marketing channel will also be piloted. For the policies and practices component, the school nutrition needs assessment will be conducted and the information shared with interested school stakeholders. The pilot will not, however, involve convening a new school wellness council or actively engaging with school stakeholders in working toward policy and practice change. The data collection protocol for the primary and secondary outcomes and process data will be piloted. Piloting the nutrition needs assessment for the policy and practice component will require a number of data collection forms. These include a form to collect beverage options and prices of options in vending machines, school stores, and on à la carte lines; forms to collect data on the availability and accessibility of water throughout the school; instructions for coding existing school policies related to beverage options in the school and beverage consumption for students and staff on school grounds; an interview schedule for school administration and school food service on practices and unwritten policies related to beverage availability on school ground; and a template for how the data will be summarized for school stakeholders.

Materials and Training Needs

Information on the material needs is found in the logic model created as part of Step 7 (see Chapter 4). The materials required for the classroom curriculum include peer leader and teacher guides and all relevant training materials, as well as any materials such as props for stations activities and related student worksheets. The materials for the social media campaign include any text, pictures, or videos to be included in Facebook or Instagram pages as well as scripts to be used for intercom messages and posters to be displayed in the hallways. The materials required for the policy and practice component include the data collection forms for the school needs assessment and the template for displaying school-specific data from the needs assessment. In addition, a template for meetings logs and minutes should be created.

For the Healthy Teens, Health Planet intervention, training needs are limited to training teachers and peer leaders to deliver the curriculum. For the classroom curriculum component, teachers and peer leaders will be trained at the same time. As a group, the teachers and peer leaders will receive a brief overview of the importance of this topic, how the formative assessment informed this intervention, and a brief explanation of why it is important to follow and adhere to the protocol. Next, teachers and peer leaders will receive an overview of the three components and will be led through the teacher and peer leader manuals to see the learning objectives and materials needed for each session. The teachers and peer leaders will then be separated, and the peer leaders trained on how to implement the two peer-led station activities. Meanwhile, the teachers will receive training on how to coordinate and oversee the group project, and how to support the peer leaders during each session, and how to complete the process evaluation checklist at the end of each session. When they are brought back together, the peer leaders practice leading both sessions with the teachers acting as students in the class and the teachers practice explaining the group project to the students.

At the end of the pilot phase, the intervention team reviews all process data, meets with relevant stakeholders to get their feedback on the pilot, and, if necessary, conducts additional formative work to understand the improvements and changes that are necessary. Any changes made to the intervention and related materials are documented in the IMOP.

SUMMARY OF THE IMPLEMENT PHASE

The two steps in the Implement Phase are crucial to the design of an effective intervention. Process data are essential to understand how the intervention worked and for finalizing all protocol, materials, and training; testing it in a pilot represents the culmination of the design process to this point. These steps are also essential for documenting what occurred in the intervention—things both planned and unplanned—and how they influenced behavioral outcomes. This information is required for full transparency as to what occurred in the intervention, to guide future revisions and adaptations, and to increase the translation and dissemination of the intervention to other communities. At the end of this phase, the team is ready to conduct a full evaluation of the intervention.

6

The Evaluate Phase

In this chapter on the Evaluate Phase, I attempt to bridge the differences between practitioners who are evaluating the success of programs in their communities and behavioral scientists conducting rigorous intervention trials. I provide basic information on planning evaluations from a practitioner's perspective as well as a heads-up for complex evaluation issues that are important for the behavioral scientist on a team to know and conceptually understand. All of the intricacies and details of evaluation methods would be too much to cover in this chapter and would involve complexities that extend beyond my expertise. There are many excellent sources for both basic evaluation methods and those specific to multilevel interventions (MLIs; Centers for Disease Control and Prevention [CDC], 2011; Grembowski, 2016; Humphrey & LeBreton, 2019; Murray, 1998; Shadish et al., 2002).

The first four sections of this chapter focus on considerations for Step 11: "Evaluate the effectiveness of the intervention." The first section provides a brief overview of the basics of program evaluation and discusses the steps and types of evaluation, important elements of study design, and threats to internal and external validity. The second section drills down to a more comprehensive discussion about measurement issues that are key to evaluating interventions, with an emphasis on understanding the importance of using valid and reliable measurement tools to assess determinants from multiple levels of influence. The third section covers evaluating the conceptual model used in designing the intervention, specifically, examining potential mediators and moderators of the

https://doi.org/10.1037/0000292-007
Designing Interventions to Promote Community Health: A Multilevel, Stepwise Approach,
by L. A. Lytle

intervention effect. The fourth section highlights issues to be aware of with the design and analysis of group- or cluster-randomized trials. The final section of this chapter focuses on Step 12: "Prepare for the next iteration or dissemination of the intervention." It includes a discussion of considerations related to examining change and maintenance of change in intervention efforts and presents a call for studying the long-term impact of behavior change interventions at both the individual and systems levels.

The final two steps in the design process are as follows:

11. Evaluate the effectiveness of the intervention
12. Prepare for the next iteration or dissemination of the intervention

STEP 11: EVALUATE THE EFFECTIVENESS OF THE INTERVENTION

Overview of Program Evaluation

Distinctions have been made between the intent of intervention research versus program evaluation, but these distinctions are beginning to blur (CDC, 2011). Traditionally, behavioral intervention research has focused on testing hypotheses using highly controlled experiments, with an end goal of advancing knowledge, while the intent of program evaluation has been to inform and improve specific community-based programs and practices. Typically, academicians report the results of their experiments to other academicians and policy makers through published research, while practitioners translate their findings to a wide set of stakeholders using a variety of communication channels. But the dichotomy between intervention research and program evaluation is actually not so distinct. Intervention research using a community-engaged approach requires that the community is involved in the design of the intervention and evaluation and is a direct and proximal beneficiary of the intervention and its findings. Likewise, community-based programs directed by public health practitioners are increasingly called on to provide evidence that their programs are effective; funders and other stakeholders want to know whether money spent on programming is making the difference it was intended to make (CDC, 2011). Therefore, both practitioners and researchers need to address evaluation as an important phase in designing MLIs to promote community health.

Steps of Evaluation

The CDC (2011) defined *program evaluation* as "the systematic collection of information about the activities, characteristics, and outcomes of programs to make judgments about the program, improve program effectiveness, and/or inform decisions about future program development" (p. 3) and suggested that there are six steps of evaluation:

1. Engage stakeholders
2. Describe the program
3. Focus the evaluation design

4. Gather credible evidence
5. Justify the conclusion
6. Ensure use of evaluation findings and share lessons learned

The first step of engaging stakeholders is built into each phase of the intervention design process described in this volume and is just as important when planning the evaluation as it is when planning the intervention. *Stakeholders* are people or organizations who are invested in what will be done through the program and with the results of the evaluation. Input from stakeholders is essential to ensure that evaluation approaches are appropriate and that the evaluation will answer questions that are important to the community. Stakeholders can be involved in many ways, including identifying and recruiting groups and individuals to be involved in the study, identifying appropriate data collection sites and methods, helping to involve community members in the evaluation team as a way to build community capacity, and interpreting study results. In addition, stakeholders who are involved in the process and recognized and respected as important team members are much more likely to be ready to act on the study's results and recommendations (Stevens et al., 2017). Without the right stakeholders involved, the program and its evaluation could be ignored, criticized, resisted, or even sabotaged.

The second step of program evaluation as conceptualized by the CDC is describing the program. This step includes work that is conducted in the Plan and Create Phases and includes developing a conceptual model and a logic model that clearly state the short, intermediate, and long-term goals and outcomes to be achieved by the intervention. Steps 3 and 4 ("Focus the evaluation design" and "Gather credible evidence") involve the primary work of the evaluation team and include choosing the most appropriate study design, measurement methods, and instruments and developing an evaluation protocol that can be delivered consistently and with rigor. This work includes creating an evaluation plan that is practical, feasible, and can be conducted within the confines of available resources and time. It is easy to overreach when making decisions about what to include in evaluation plans, but more is not necessarily better. Every aspect of the evaluation plan comes with costs including those related to

- identifying or creating and testing measurement instruments;
- training and certifying data collectors;
- software and programming expenses;
- data collection, including staff time, materials, and equipment;
- data entry, cleaning, and analysis;
- incentives for participating in evaluation activities; and
- participant burden including time, convenience, and hassle.

The quality of data collected should not be compromised by the quantity of data collected. All evaluation should be conducted in an ethical manner and produce findings that are accurate and useful to stakeholders in making decisions about program implementation, improving program effectiveness, and identifying future research and program needs.

Steps 5 and 6 involve analyzing results and reporting findings. Beyond data analysis and writing academic research papers, these steps include explaining the results to stakeholders using formats that are most useful to their purpose. It is important that evaluations serve to inform the next iteration of the intervention to improve impact or enhance its dissemination (Step 12 of the design process).

Building an Evaluation Team

Just as the team designing the intervention requires people with special skills, the team assembled to design and execute the evaluation also needs special skills. Importantly, people collecting the data should not be the same people responsible for delivering the intervention, particularly data collection that occurs during or after the end of the intervention. Once the intervention begins, the participants will likely know, or at least recognize, the interventionists with whom they have been working. Because of that association, participants' responses to evaluation questions might be biased because they may want to please the interventionist by providing the expected or "right" answer.

The evaluation team should include or be in close contact with the project lead or the principal investigator of the study and at least one program or research staff who has been engaged with all aspects of the intervention design. Evaluation staff need to understand the big picture of the intervention; this knowledge will help them make good decisions when questions of priorities come up. The team should include external stakeholders who can provide a community perspective on the evaluation plans, including issues of timing, data collection protocol, measurement tools, and staffing. The team might also need to engage consultants or contractors for evaluation aspects that require specific expertise, such as cleaning and analyzing accelerometry and diet recall data or evaluating aspects of the environment using geographical information system (GIS) software. The team will also need someone trained in and experienced with biostatistical methods. Those people may come from a variety of fields, including biostatistics, epidemiology, psychology, sociology, and others. Biostatistical expertise is required for data reduction needs, evaluating the relationships of variables within the conceptual model, and modeling and testing the effectiveness of the intervention. Multilevel trials require biostatisticians with specific expertise in analyzing group- or cluster-randomized trials.

Careful attention needs to be paid to finding the right person to be the evaluation team leader or coordinator. This individual needs to be detail oriented and very organized, as well as innovative in finding solutions to evaluation-related challenges. The evaluation team leader needs to understand the project goals, recognize potential threats to data quality, and have good insight into and respect for stakeholder interests. They also need to be able to work efficiently, effectively, and compassionately with a wide variety of stakeholders and have excellent communication skills.

The CDC identified five different types of evaluation including process evaluation which they refer to as "Implementation" and evaluation related to effectiveness, efficiency, cost effectiveness, and attribution. The type of

TYPES OF EVALUATION

The CDC (2011) specified five types of evaluation that are expected to answer the following questions:

- **Implementation:** Were the program's activities delivered as intended?
- **Effectiveness:** Did the program achieve the goals and objectives it was intended to accomplish?
- **Efficiency:** Were the program activities produced with appropriate use of budget and staff time?
- **Cost-effectiveness:** Does the value of achieving the program goals exceed the cost of achieving them?
- **Attribution:** Can goals and objectives met be attributed to the impact of the program rather than extraneous things?

evaluation that I focus on in this design process is evaluation to assign attribution. When the goal is to design a community-engaged MLI, the primary evaluation focus is on determining, with some level of confidence that behavioral changes seen at the end of the evaluation are caused by the intervention efforts. Establishing that causal relationship is challenging because a variety of factors may influence intervention targets or behavior but have little or nothing to do with the intervention. The next sections discuss some of the issues related to determining if the intervention was responsible for the behavior change.

Threats to Internal Validity

Being able to assign attribution requires study designs, measurement tools and methods, and analysis plans that reduce the risk of three types of errors. Type I error occurs when an intervention is deemed to be effective in creating change when the change actually occurred by chance. Type II error occurs when an intervention is deemed to be ineffective in creating change when actually it was effective. Type III error occurs when the intervention was not implemented as planned; this type of error is primarily identified through process evaluation. Type I and Type II errors can be minimized through appropriate study design and adequate sample size. Type III errors are minimized through careful planning, creating, and implementing of interventions.

Type I and Type II errors may occur because of threats to internal validity representing the extent to which one can be confident that behavior change can be attributed to the intervention. Three conditions must occur to establish causality between the intervention (represented analytically as the treatment variable or independent variable) and the outcome of interest (represented analytically as the dependent variable): (a) they must change together, (b) the delivery of the intervention must precede the outcome, and (c) no other factors can explain the results. The criteria of changing together does not stipulate the direction of change. The relationship between the independent and dependent variable can be in the same direction (i.e., more social support is related to increased levels of activity) or in an inverse direction (i.e., more social support is related to decreased smoking rates), but the variables must move together in a consistent pattern of change. The criteria of having the intervention precede the outcome points out the limitations of cross-sectional study designs. If the determinants of the behavior targeted through intervention strategies and the behavior are measured at the same time, attribution of the behavioral outcome to the intervention cannot be made; an association may be evident, but causality cannot be determined. The third requirement is that no other factors, also referred to as confounders or extraneous factors, can explain the results of the study. Confounders are discussed in a following section.

There are eight threats to internal validity that can result in misattribution of cause and effect: history, maturation, instrumentation, testing, selection bias, regression to the mean, contamination, and attrition. Table 6.1 provides a definition of each threat and an example of how it may occur in a study. Threats to internal validity are conditions or occurrences that may happen before, during, or after an intervention that influence the outcome or dependent variable but are not related to any intervention efforts. Attention to study design and analytic strategies can help mitigate the impact of threats to internal validity.

Study Designs

A randomized controlled trial (RCT) is the gold standard for establishing attribution or causality. An RCT involves recruiting a sample to participate in the study (the sample could be units representing individuals, groups, or even communities), collecting baseline measures on the sample (those measures include the outcome of interest and other variables represented in the conceptual model), and then randomly assigning units to intervention and control conditions. Those randomized to the intervention condition receive the intervention, while those in the control group do not; at the end of the intervention period, both intervention and control groups participate in postintervention measures. The effectiveness of the intervention is determined by the difference in the behavior between groups at the follow-up period either by comparing the difference in behavior change between groups from baseline to postintervention or by comparing the groups' behavior postintervention, controlling for baseline levels of behavior. The hypothesis being evaluated is that units randomized to the intervention group will experience greater change in the targeted outcome postintervention period compared with those randomized to the control group.

Randomization is important because it controls for both known and unknown confounding factors. Confounding factors are characteristics of the sample that may be associated with both the behavioral outcome (the dependent variable) and the intervention and determinants that the intervention is trying to influence (the independent variables). Common confounders at the individual level may include age, sex, and education. Other types of confounders may exist for groups randomized to treatment conditions, such as size of the organization or the proportion of the community living below poverty levels. Failing to account for confounding can result in misattribution of the effect of the intervention.

TABLE 6.1. Threats to Internal Validity: Definitions and Examples

Type of threat	Definition	Example
History	An unrelated event happening in the larger environment influences the results of the study	A national campaign to increase the public's awareness of the importance of colorectal screening is launched in the middle of a regional colon screening intervention.
Maturation (secular)	The outcomes of the study vary as a natural result of time	Change in body weight is being considered as the dependent variable in a weight gain prevention study with youth, but youth will naturally gain weight over time.
Instrumentation	Different measures are used at different time points	A "better" audit tool for assessing the retail store environment is discovered after baseline data were collected using a different audit tool.
Testing	The experience of taking the test (survey) influences future responses	Workers' awareness of sexual harassment in the workplace is asked about in a survey. The follow-up survey assessing awareness will reflect the workers' experience from taking the baseline survey.
Selection bias	Groups are not comparable at the beginning of the study	A quasi-experimental design is used assigning communities to intervention or comparison groups. At baseline, the communities differ by important characteristics, including median income and unemployment rates.
Regression to the mean	Exceptionally high or low values at baseline will move closer to the middle over time	Those with the highest blood pressure at baseline are likely to have a lower blood pressure reading in a follow-up measurement period.
Contamination (social interaction)	Participants assigned to different groups interact with each other	An intervention is launched using a social media site but there are no controls for keeping those randomized to the control condition from the site.
Attrition	Participants or units drop out of the study	20 community centers agree to participate in a randomized control trial. Half of those centers randomized to the control condition drop out upon hearing their assignment.

Randomization is the most robust way to ensure equivalency of groups at baseline and to avoid threats to internal validity (Cleary et al., 2012; Murray et al., 2010).

Simple randomization occurs when individual units are randomly assigned to either the intervention or control condition using a random numbers table or some other method of random assignment. Blocking, also called stratification, may be used when there is a concern that potential confounders may not be distributed equally between the two conditions. Before randomization, the units are placed in groups (or blocks) by the presence or absence of confounders, and randomization is done such that units are assigned equally across conditions. Blocking or stratification should be limited to those factors known to be significantly related to both the treatment and the outcome. Blocking on too many characteristics may threaten randomization by influencing the distribution of unknown confounders.

MLIs use other study designs to promote population health, but they come with important limitations. Quasi-experimental study designs involve comparing the effectiveness of an intervention between two groups without randomization. The study team decides the assignment of group to condition, and the conditions are called the intervention and comparison (rather than control) groups. There may be an attempt to reduce the introduction of confounders by matching the groups on key characteristics, but it is difficult to identify all the potential characteristics on which to match. Because of the potential for non-equivalent groups at baseline, a quasi-experimental design is not as robust for establishing causality as an RCT. But sometimes, particularly with interventions that occur at the level of community or other large systems, randomization is not possible, and a well-designed and conducted quasi-experimental study may be the best option (Cleary et al., 2012; Murray et al., 2010).

Natural experiments are another example of a quasi-experimental study. The introduction of some change in a community that is not part of a planned program or intervention trial provides an opportunity to examine the effects of that change on aspects of health behavior. As examples, a citywide policy on foods available in convenience stores, a state-wide tax on sugar-sweetened beverages (SSBs), the introduction of a full-service grocery store in a food desert, or the addition of sidewalks and additional green space in a neighborhood may be expected to influence the health behavior of people living in those communities. With natural experiments, randomization is obviously not possible, but often a comparison community is chosen and a study is designed to collect data from individuals in both communities as a way to examine the impact of the change. As with other nonrandomized designs, nonequivalence of the groups at baseline poses the biggest threat to internal validity. Study designs using only two communities will not be able to examine causality because it is nearly impossible to disentangle the effect of the intervention from existing differences between two communities (Murray et al., 2010).

A single-condition, pre–post study design may be helpful in a pilot phase to provide some estimate of the potential for the intervention to lead to change. Without a comparison group, however, a pre–post design can show progress toward a goal but cannot attribute the change seen between the beginning and end of the intervention to the intervention. Many things might happen between baseline and the end of the intervention, resulting in a change in the outcome that is unrelated to the intervention (Cleary et al., 2012; Murray et al., 2010).

External Validity

External validity refers to the extent to which one can generalize the findings of a study to other settings or groups. Findings from an intervention study that has restrictive inclusion criteria may not generalize to the same intervention

AN ILLUSTRATION OF THE IMPORTANCE OF THE STUDY DESIGN IN ESTABLISHING ATTRIBUTION

Consider a church-based intervention designed to help parishioners control their hypertension. The intervention will include group classes on managing hypertension through stress reduction techniques and low-sodium cooking classes. The outcomes to be assessed include two behavioral measures (sodium intake and behaviors related to stress management) and a biological outcome (blood pressure). The proposed study design is that the first 20 people to meet eligibility criteria and sign up for the study will get the intervention and the next 20 people will be the comparison group. The outcomes will be evaluated by assessing the difference in the baseline and follow-up measures between the intervention and comparison groups.

The lack of randomization to condition poses several threats to internal validity. Those who signed up first may be especially interested in the class because their hypertension is not well-controlled, resulting in the baseline blood pressure levels being higher in the intervention compared with the comparison group. That baseline difference may affect how blood pressure levels change over time but have little to do with the impact of the intervention; this is an example of the threat to internal validity *regression to the mean*. In addition, it might be that the first to hear about the study were women from a senior Bible study group. Those women and friends they contacted about the study will likely end up in the intervention group because they heard about the study first. As a result, the two treatment groups may differ by age and sex at baseline, resulting in *selection bias*.

In this example, attribution of the intervention to the outcome would be enhanced if the 40 people who expressed interest in the study and met eligibility criteria were randomly assigned to condition after baseline data collection. Blocking may also be used to distribute potential confounders equally between the treatment groups, such as severity of hypertension, gender, and age.

conducted in other samples. Think of study conducted with a sample restricted to boys attending private schools; results and conclusions from that study may not apply very well to a general school population. Likewise, interventions that rely on the unique expertise or skills of individuals delivering the intervention may not be generalizable to other settings because replicating that expertise would be unlikely. Think of hiring a celebrity to deliver aspects of an intervention; the intervention may result in positive changes, but scaling up that approach to other communities may be difficult.

External validity will always be somewhat limited in community-engaged health behavior interventions because they are designed to influence the behavioral determinants relevant to a specific community. That tailoring of determinants helps increase the chance that the intervention will be effective but may limit its generalizability to other communities. Interventions that have been found to be successful in changing the target behavior in one or several other communities will likely need some adaptation for each new community. (In Chapter 7, I talk about how the intervention design process can be used to adapt existing interventions.) At the same time, intervention approaches and strategies employed to make an impact on a determinant should be designed to have a broad application that is useful in many communities (Glasgow et al., 2003).

CONSORT Guidelines for Evaluating the Quality of a Study

A study team conducting an RCT may be asked to complete a CONSORT diagram and checklist for its study. CONSORT, which stands for Consolidating Standards of Reporting Trials, was developed in the mid-1990s by an international group of investigators conducting clinical trials, statisticians, epidemiologists, and editors of biomedical journals (Begg et al., 1996). The purpose of CONSORT is to provide specific information about the design, context, conduct, analysis, results, and interpretation of an RCT, allowing for assessment of the study's quality. Sometimes this diagram and checklist need to be completed to fulfill some requirement of a funder; in other cases, use of the CONSORT process is required as part of the publication process. In either case, attention to the CONSORT approach helps a research team attend to potential threats to study quality and be as transparent as possible in presenting study results. Elements of the intervention are also to be addressed through the CONSORT process and are specified in a checklist (Moher et al., 2001). Figure 6.1 shows the flow diagram to be completed as part of the CONSORT process and includes information on enrollment, allocation to treatment, follow-up, and analysis. A version of CONSORT with specific considerations for group- or cluster-randomized trials, including MLIs, was published in 2012 (Campbell et al., 2012).

Montgomery et al. (2018) examined the CONSORT process and made recommendations for improving how social and psychosocial interventions (SPIs) are reported in the literature. They noted that descriptions of RCTs evaluating behavioral trials are often "insufficiently accurate, comprehensive, and transparent to replicate trials, assess their quality, and understand for whom and under what circumstances an intervention should be delivered" (p. 2). They highlighted the lack of intervention detail included in most outcome papers reporting on RCTs, including the specific techniques used to change behavior, the materials used, how the intervention was implemented, how the providers were trained, and any adaptations done to existing interventions. Montgomery and colleagues also noted how infrequently information on the involvement of community stakeholders is included in study descriptions. They suggested that this lack of transparency is likely the cause of suboptimal dissemination of effective interventions.

Montgomery and colleagues (2018) recommended using the CONSORT-SPI 2018 extension that asks for additional information specific to the intervention, including:

- how the intervention was hypothesized to work
- specification of the unit of randomization and analysis

FIGURE 6.1. CONSORT Diagram

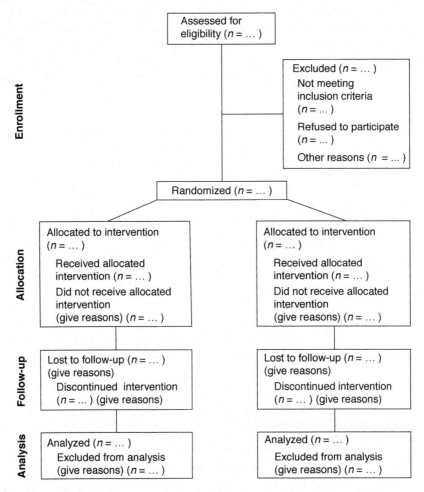

Note. CONSORT = Consolidating Standards of Reporting Trials. From "The CONSORT Statement: Revised Recommendations for Improving the Quality of Reports of Parallel Group Randomized Trials," by D. Moher, K. F. Schulz, and D. G. Altman, 2001, *BMC Medical Research Methodology*, *1*(Article 2), p. 5 (https://doi.org/10.1186/1471-2288-1-2). Copyright 2001 by D. Moher, K. F. Schulz, and D. G. Altman. Adapted with permission.

- eligibility criteria for intervention settings and those delivering the intervention
- extent to which the intervention as planned was delivered and received by participants
- where other informational materials about delivering the intervention can be accessed
- how intervention providers were assigned to groups
- information on intervention developer and stakeholder involvement in the trial design, conduct, or analysis
- incentives offered as part of the trial

Montgomery et al. (2018) suggested that in addition to funders and publishers, there are other stakeholders who would find the revised CONSORT diagram and checklist helpful, including the study designers as they consider ways to ensure the quality of their studies, as well as policy makers and practitioners who can use these guidelines to help identify and implement effective interventions for specific communities. The TIDieR (Template for Intervention Description and Replication) checklist mentioned in Chapter 5 of this volume is yet another extension of this effort to make the details of the intervention more transparent and it is a product of the international Equator Network (Enhancing the Quality and Transparency of Health Research; http://equator-network.org). The goal of Equator is to improve the reliability and value of published health research literature by promoting transparent and accurate reporting.

Measurement Issues With MLIs

To evaluate the effectiveness of MLIs, the team must be able to assess change in the determinants chosen as the focus of the intervention as well as the behavior targeted for change. With MLIs, this means that the team will need to assess determinants from the individual environment, such as attitudes, beliefs, and perceptions; determinants from the social environment, including normative behaviors, social networks, and social support; and determinants

WHY SHOULD PRACTITIONERS CARE ABOUT REPORTING GUIDELINES?

Practitioners may not intend to publish the findings of their program evaluation in a scientific publication or present results at a scientific meeting. The emphasis of their evaluation may be more pragmatic, with a focus more on how the intervention worked in their specific community and less on scientific rigor. They may not intend to try to disseminate their intervention broadly. Still, details of how an intervention works help to inform best practices for public health.

Being aware of the types of issues that are considered in evaluating the impact of an intervention and being clear about the limitations of program evaluation efforts are both essential to interpreting the study's findings and making recommendations about next steps. Likewise, a practitioner may never be asked to complete a TIDieR checklist to provide full transparency of their intervention to community stakeholders, but such checklists may serve as a reminder of the details that will be needed for another community group to adapt or adopt the intervention. All evaluation and reporting work should have goals to increase transparency about what was attempted and achieved in a project, advance knowledge about what worked and what did not, and disseminate best practices to help inform other community health promotion efforts.

from the physical environment, including access, availability, cues, and reinforcement. All of the tools chosen should demonstrate some measure of validity and reliability. Poorly measured determinants add error and sometimes systematic bias to the analyses. This bias may invalidate the results, threatening the conclusions that can be made about studies. In this section, I describe the challenges faced in measuring health behaviors and how the concepts of validity and reliability are applied to behaviors and determinants across the individual, social, and physical environments.

Measuring Health Behavior
The attributes that the behavioral sciences attempt to measure differ from those attributes measured in the biological sciences. Many measurement tools available to the biological sciences provide a direct measure of health risk. Think of taking a blood sample to assess serum blood cholesterol or using a sphygmomanometer to take blood pressure; those measures provide an objective assessment of an individual's risk for disease.

While some behaviors pose demonstrable and significant health risk (Dwyer-Lindgren et al., 2017), assessing health behaviors poses significant challenges. Many health behaviors are private (i.e., sleep, sexual activity, hygiene). Some health behaviors are intermittent (i.e., health screenings, vaccinations, dental checkups), while other health behaviors occur many times each day (i.e., eating, activity, screen time). Some health behaviors incur risk only in high doses over an extended period of time (i.e., high fat intake or persistent sleep deprivation), while other behaviors are risky in any frequency or dose (i.e., driving while under the influence of alcohol or the use of tobacco products). Many behavioral patterns happen in clusters or covary with other behaviors, making it difficult to attribute risk to a specific behavior (Lytle et al., 1995). The measurement of many, if not most, health behaviors relies on self-report. All of these factors make it exceedingly difficult to measure health behaviors in an objective and nonbiased manner.

In some cases, biomarkers can be used to assess health behavior. A *biomarker* is an objective indication of a biological state that does not rely on self-report and can be measured accurately and reproducibly (Strimbu & Tavel, 2010). For example, a urine test for cotinine can determine whether an individual has been exposed to nicotine. Likewise, the use of doubly labeled water from blood, urine, or saliva samples can be used as a marker for energy intake, and urinary nitrogen can be used to measure protein intake (Potischman & Freudenheim, 2003). Biomarkers are often used as the gold standard for showing a biological consequence of a behavior and are useful in the early epidemiologic research phase linking the behavior with disease risk. However, the use of biomarkers as a way to measure behavior is usually not feasible in fully powered, community-engaged behavior change interventions. The requirements and expenses related to obtaining and processing a sample of blood, urine, or saliva or other biomarkers are often out of reach for interventions that are being evaluated in a community setting. In addition, the external validity of the behavioral estimates based on the use of biomarkers will be limited; the behavioral estimates from individuals who are willing to provide biological specimens for a research trial or spend time in clinical settings as part of a measurement protocol may not generalize to the behavior in the larger population.

Most community-based interventions need to rely on self-report to assess behavior. Self-report data are replete with the potential for error and bias. As an example, in using a 24-hour recall to assess dietary intake, the team faces the challenges of memory (Does the individual remember everything that they ate in the past 24 hours?), estimation (Can the individual estimate serving sizes consumed?), knowledge (Does the individual know if ground turkey or pork was used in the stew served at a friend's house?), and embarrassment (Does the individual want to admit to eating a pint of ice cream before bedtime?). In addition to these challenges, the team may need to distinguish between typical versus unusual behavior. For example, using a single 24-hour recall to measure some aspect of eating behavior risks that the recall does not represent usual intake; think about the information collected from a dietary recall taken the day after Halloween or on a Saturday versus a Tuesday. If the team uses a dietary screener instead, asking individuals to report on their usual intake of candy, fruits, vegetables, or processed foods over the past month or past year, they face new challenges, including the individual's ability to estimate food consumption over a long period of time and group foods into categories. Although some of this bias will be random and is likely to occur equally across groups, other bias is systematic and more likely to occur in some groups than in others. As an example, those with obesity have been found to be more likely to substantially underreport dietary intake, especially energy intake, compared with those without obesity (Schoeller, 1995), representing systematic bias. Systematic bias increases the chances that the conclusions drawn from the data will be flawed.

Self-report provides a relative estimate of behavior that is useful for ranking or grouping individuals along some risk continuum compared with more objective methods that provide a direct and accurate measure of an individual's risk. This is an important distinction between measurement used in public or population health compared with measures used to estimate individual clinical outcomes. As an example, the use of a fruit and vegetable screener to assess an individual's risk for colon cancer would be a poor predictor of risk. Many other factors will need to be considered before the individual's cancer risk can be determined, including other behaviors they engage in, preexisting conditions, an assessment of biomarkers to identify genetic factors, and an assessment of other exposures to carcinogens. However, a self-report screener to estimate a group's average intake of fruits and vegetables can be used in public health surveillance to estimate population-level risk or to evaluate the effectiveness of a community-based intervention. Although there will be error in the self-report measure used, the measurement error is spread over individuals within each group, providing a more stable estimate of group-level behavior. As such, it is appropriate to compare behavior change between those randomized to an intervention or control group, disease risk in males versus females, or smokers versus nonsmokers.

The assessment of physical activity (PA), sedentary behavior, and sleep patterns through the use of actigraphy stands as an exception to the inherent difficulties of measuring behavior. Objective counts of movement can be obtained through actigraphy; an individual is asked to wear a device on their wrist, ankle, or thigh for a given amount of time each day, for a set number of days. Movement is monitored and data captured through the actigraph. Unlike pedometers or other activity monitors that allow the individual to see step counts or activity throughout the day, actigraphy data are not available to the individual, minimizing the likelihood that seeing their activity levels will influence their behavior. Actigraphs can also be worn at night to assess the amount and patterns of sleep. Because self-report is not required, a more objective assessment of the behavior is possible. Measurement error is still an issue; individuals may forget to wear the actigraph or increase their activity in response to wearing a device. Errors may occur as part of downloading or analyzing the data. Still, several sources of potential error are eliminated by not relying on self-report.

Measuring the Determinants of Behavior

When evaluating the effectiveness of MLIs, it is important to measure the determinants that are targeted through the intervention strategies. If the intervention was not successful in positively influencing the determinants targeted, it is unlikely that it will be successful in achieving health outcomes. This information is extremely helpful in understanding how the intervention worked and the components that were particularly successful, or unsuccessful, in changing behavior. With this information, the team is better able to revise their intervention and make it stronger.

Determinants from the three environments I have discussed throughout this design process (the individual, social, and physical environments) are often measured in different ways. A reminder about nomenclature may be helpful: Determinants are similar to theoretical constructs and are represented in the conceptual model. After data collection, cleaning, and reduction, these determinants become variables to be used in data analysis. The most common data collection tools for constructs representing the individual environment are surveys and questionnaires. Often, a set of questions is developed to represent a single determinant or construct; for example, a set of questions is developed to assess self-efficacy for a behavioral response. Most often, those questions are reduced into a single variable using a data reduction technique, such as creating a scale or an index.

The social environment may be assessed through behavioral surveys of the important referents of the sample as a way to determine the extent to which role modeling or observational learning occurs. As an example, to assess the extent to which smoking behavior is modeled in a worksite, a survey that assesses smoking behavior of workers may be conducted, and the proportion of workers who smoke at work may be used as a variable representing role modeling. Social network analysis and dyadic analysis are other measurement methods to assess the social environment. Social network analysis attempts to quantify the number and strength of social connections between groups of individuals to understand how those networks affect the health and behaviors of individuals within the network (Valente, 2015). Dyadic analysis occurs when identical data are collected for dyads (e.g., parent and child, two friends). The data analysis is designed to examine the extent to which an individual and their dyadic partner have an effect on the outcome of interest (e.g., a health behavior, health outcome), either simultaneously or independently. The actor partner interdependence model is the most widely used analytic model of dyadic data in the epidemiologic literature (Kenny et al., 2020). For both social network analysis and dyadic analysis, data are collected from individuals using self-report surveys or some objectively measured health outcome, such as HIV infection or body weight. Conducting social network or dyadic analysis requires significant advance planning and hypotheses that are considered before the study begins. In addition, expertise in analyzing and interpreting these types of data is needed.

Assessing the physical environment may include the use of audits and observational tools created specifically for that purpose. These tools may be developed to be used by trained staff or by study participants. As examples, an observation form may be developed to evaluate the user-friendliness or a neighborhood's walkability. Data collectors are trained to use a form to document information on such things as presence of sidewalks, cleanliness, lighting, or graffiti on buildings (Sallis et al., 2010). As another example, a data collection form might be developed for parents to document the foods available in their home (Fulkerson et al., 2008). GIS is used to assess features of a neighborhood physical environment. This system integrates and analyzes geographic data derived from existing databases that have a spatial reference, or are "geolocated," such as U.S. Census data linked to census track and block groups. Using that spatial data to define the area of interest, other data sources are linked to those areas to provide information on the availability and accessibility of health-promoting or health-compromising environmental elements. For example, GIS can be used to document the availability of foods in a geographic area by linking the spatial data with other data sources that document the existence and types of food outlets in that area. GIS can also be used with other citywide data that show how communities may differ in the availability of park and recreation areas or how street connectivity and density may influence residents' ability to walk for transportation or leisure. Other existing measures that might be used to represent the physical environment may include store licensing data and sales data or the number and promotional messages found on billboards or in store windows (Lytle, 2009). Using GIS in a study requires a team member with specific expertise in using geographic and spatial analysis software.

Identifying Reliable and Valid Measurement Tools

Choosing the most robust measurement tools possible is an extremely important evaluation task. For measurement tools, that "robustness" is assessed primarily by showing that the tool used is both reliable and valid. *Reliability* refers to the measure's consistency, and *validity* refers to the measure's ability to assess what is intended to be measured. The field of psychology has long paid attention to the psychometric properties of measures used to assess abstract concepts such as attitudes and beliefs. In addition, measurement tools and methods used to assess behavior have typically relied on estimates of reliability and validity to

MEASURING SOCIAL DETERMINANTS OF HEALTH AND EVALUATION WITH AN EQUITY LENS

Social determinants of health (SDOH)—defined by the World Health Organization as the conditions in which people are born, grow, live, work, and age, which are shaped by the distribution of money, power, and resources—are well-recognized as factors that have direct and complex effects on health. Although MLIs are not resourced to directly intervene on SDOH, measuring and documenting SDOH's impact on population health is an important step in identifying holistic strategies to promote health and well-being of communities.

The work of identifying measurement tools to be used to assess SDOH is underway. A review of the literature by Elias et al. (2019) showed that the SDOH tools meeting review criteria spanned three broad categories: (a) health—surveillance tools to document the health of populations; (b) built environment—tools created for neighborhood needs assessment that assess urban planning, community development, economic development, and public policy; and (c) cross-sectoral—tools that combine both health and built environment data for the purpose of needs assessment, surveillance, and evaluation. Unfortunately, the review showed little consensus on the specific indicators or questions that are used to measure these broad categories. The lack of agreement on how to measure important SDOH, including basic indicators such as employment, income equality, and poverty levels in a community, will make it difficult to compare findings across studies. Work to standardize measurement tools is needed.

The movement to better understand and address SDOH must include approaching evaluation with an equity lens. Work by Public Policy Associates (2015) addresses the inherent limitations of conducting an evaluation in a community when the evaluators have limited understanding of the communities they are trying to serve, fail to engage in deep listening to the community, and do not attempt to assess diversity, inclusion, and equity concerns that exists in the community. Public Policy Associates (2015) developed a resource, "Considerations for Conducting Evaluation Using a Culturally Responsive and Racial Equity Lens," as a practical guide to conducting evaluation using an equity lens. The resource includes advice on how to assemble more culturally competent measurement teams; craft more culturally responsive evaluation designs; gather valuable perspectives from groups that have been silent, ignored, or misunderstood; and increase understanding of the reach, effectiveness, and impact of community-based interventions and programs.

Even though the individual programs and interventions that we design may not be able to directly influence the deep causes of health disparities, being intentional about how our evaluation efforts can be used to reflect the realities of communities, document health inequities, and contribute to a more inclusive society is an important goal.

show the relationship between self-report measures and more objective measures of behavior. However, the importance of the psychometric properties of tools to estimate the physical environment is just beginning to be appreciated (Lytle, 2009; Lytle & Sokol, 2017).

There are three primary types of reliability to consider: interrater reliability, test–retest reliability, and internal consistency.

Interrater reliability evaluates the degree to which data collected by two independent data collectors are consistent. Interrater reliability does not apply to self-report measures, only to measurements that are taken by a data collector observing some phenomena. Interrater reliability is relevant to measures taken to represent the physical environment, such as audits of foods in a store or the cleanliness of neighborhood parks and recreation areas. As examples, two independent data collectors who are gathering data on the availability of fruits and vegetables in a corner store at the same time should be collecting concordant data. Lack of agreement typically suggests that the data collection form or protocol is not clear or that data collectors have not been adequately trained. Interrater reliability would also be relevant if data on social interactions were obtained

TYPES OF RELIABILITY AND VALIDITY

Reliability

- **Interrater reliability:** The degree to which data collected by two independent data collectors are consistent

- **Test–retest reliability:** The extent to which measurements that are taken at two time periods are consistent

- **Internal consistency:** The extent to which questions designed to tap the same construct are correlated with each other

Validity

- **Face validity:** The degree to which the measurement tool appears to be measuring the construct of interest

- **Content validity:** The extent to which the measurement tool captures the full breadth of the content desired

- **Criterion validity:** The degree to which the data collected from the measurement instrument agrees with a criterion measure (or gold standard measure) of the same construct

- **Construct validity:** The extent to which the measure of interest is associated or correlated with other constructs in the conceptual model in the hypothesized direction

by having data collectors observe or listen to social interactions—for example, observing how parents interact with their children about eating behaviors at mealtime or listening to tapes of couples engaged in resolving some conflict. Two independent data collectors would use the same data collection form and protocol at the same time, and interrater reliability would be established if the data they collect were in close agreement. Agreement in the range of 0.41–0.60 using a kappa coefficient is considered fair, and agreement above 0.61 is considered moderate (Grembowski, 2016).

Test–retest reliability assesses the extent to which measurements taken at two time periods are associated. Test–retest reliability can apply to self-report data as well as data gathered by data collectors. For example, if a set of survey questions are used to assess an individual's sense of perceived control over their ability to resist the urge to smoke in high-risk situations, the individual's response to those questions should be similar, although not necessarily identical, week to week. Test–retest can also be important to establish for measures of the social and physical environments. Lower levels of test–retest for audit tools tapping the social or physical environment may suggest that the environment being observed changes over time. Imagine collecting observational data on the foods available at a farmer's market; seasonal differences by observation period are to be expected. To address collecting data on environments that are expected to change, attention should be paid to the data collection schedule and the level of detail collected. Agreement in the range of 0.41–0.60 using a kappa coefficient is considered fair, and agreement above 0.61 is considered moderate (Grembowski, 2016).

The final way that reliability is assessed is by evaluating the internal consistency of items designed to assess a construct. Often a set of questions is used to collect data on a construct, and the results of the answers are combined to create a single scale or variable used to assess the construct. For example, a set of questions is designed to assess one's perceptions of social support and includes asking about sources of social support, the ways that social support is given, and one's satisfaction with their level of social support. Internal consistency, as measured by Cronbach's alpha, confirms that the questions used are all related to the same construct—in this example, one's perceptions of social support. If internal consistency is weak (or the Cronbach's alpha is below 0.70), it may be that some of the questions are not tapping the intended construct (Nunnally, 1978). Eliminating or replacing the questions that do not hang together in the scale or are not correlated with each other will increase the scale's ability to assess change in the determinant.

There are four main types of validity to consider.

Face validity refers to the degree to which the measurement tool appears to be measuring the construct of interest. Face validity is established by having experts review the measurement questions or tool and affirming that the questions seem appropriate to their intent. As an example, a set of questions to assess perceived barriers is reviewed by a group of experts. On the basis of their review, questions that are more closely related to assessing perceived stress are eliminated from the set of questions because they are tapping into a related but unique construct. Face validity cannot be quantitatively determined because it relies on the subjective assessment of some expert or group of experts.

Content validity refers to the extent to which the measurement tool captures the full breadth of the content desired. For example, if a set of questions is developed to assess individual-level perceptions of self-efficacy for enacting a behavior, that set should include questions related to a variety of situations in which self-efficacy for the behavioral response is important. Likewise, if a data collection tool is designed to assess the accessibility of fruits and vegetables at a corner store, the tool should assess multiple aspects of accessibility, including the price, placement, and promotions related to fruits and vegetables. If the measure lacks content validity, the relationship between the determinant and outcome may be artificially low. Like face validity, content validity is most often determined through expert opinion; quantitative methods for establishing content validity are underdeveloped (Koller et al., 2017).

Criterion validity is established by examining the association or correlation between data collected using a gold standard or criterion measure and data obtained from the construct as measured. Criterion validity cannot be estimated for many psychosocial constructs, such as attitudes, beliefs, or perceptions, because there is no true criterion or gold standard for what one believes or perceives. It is more commonly used in evaluating the rigor of psychosocial measures for which a clinical standard is available or for behavioral or environmental measures. For example, some clinical assessment used to diagnose depression may be used as the gold standard to establish the criterion validity of a short survey used to assess depressive symptoms. Likewise, if self-report is used to estimate individual caloric intake, a biomarker such as doubly labeled water may be used as the criterion measure on which to judge the relative accuracy of the self-report tool. Similarly, if one is trying to estimate the availability of low-calorie snacks in a convenience store, data from an observation or audit form might be compared with the store's purchasing and sales data. Criterion validity above 0.60 is generally considered acceptable (Grembowski, 2016).

Finally, *construct validity* refers to the extent to which the measure of interest is associated or correlated with other constructs in the conceptual model in a hypothesized direction. As examples, one would expect that a variable created to assess perceived barriers to enacting a behavior would show an inverse relationship with the behavior of interest (more barriers, less behavior). Likewise, a variable created to assess perceptions of social support for a behavior should be positively related to perceptions of self-efficacy for enacting the behavior (more social support, more self-efficacy). Relationships that are counterintuitive suggest a problem with the measurement tool or variable construction. If construct validity is not established, the ability to evaluate the relationships of the constructs in a conceptual model is in question. Correlation coefficients in the range of 0.20 to 0.80 are acceptable for establishing construct validity (Drummond et al., 2016; Streiner & Norman, 2003; Swank & Mullen, 2017).

Example of Choosing Measurement Tools: Healthy Teens, Healthy Planet

For the team attempting to evaluate the effectiveness of an MLI, time and resources need to be devoted to identifying the most robust measurement tools to use. Consider the case study of Healthy Teens, Healthy Planet, a school-based intervention to reduce students' consumption of SSBs. The constructs that the team will need to assess to evaluate the effectiveness of their intervention are as follows:

- behavioral outcome: student consumption of SSBs

- determinants from the individual environment:
  - perceived control of beverage choices
  - perceived barriers to making healthy beverage choices
  - knowledge about healthy beverage choices

- determinants from the social environment:
  - observational learning/role-modeling around beverage choices at school
  - descriptive norm regarding typical beverage choice for peers
  - social reinforcement and incentives for making healthy beverage choices

- determinants from the physical environment:
  - availability of beverage options on school property
  - accessibility of beverage options on school property

For each of these constructs, the team will need to identify a measurement tool or method that will allow them to create a variable representing each construct for use in analytic models. For the team to have some assurance that the variable to be created is a good representation of the construct, the measurement tool used to collect data needs to demonstrate both reliability and validity.

To assess the behavior (the dependent variable), the team is considering using a beverage screener as a way to assess students' SSB consumption. Interrater reliability is not an issue because a self-report measurement tool will be used. However, the team would want to choose an existing screener that shows moderate levels of test–retest reliability and shows good internal consistency to be assured that the tool provides consistent results. They would also be looking for an existing screener that shows face and content validity. The team wants to confirm that the questions about beverage consumption are relevant to their population. They also look for a screener that has been evaluated against a gold standard to show that it has criterion validity (most likely multiple 24-hour recalls). Finally, evidence that the variable constructed from the screener is associated with other relevant constructs, such as body mass index or the incidence of dental caries, would provide evidence that the screener has construct validity.

The team is attempting to positively influence several determinants from the individual environment. They are looking for a measure that will represent the construct of students' perceived barriers to choosing healthy beverages at school.

Again, interrater reliability is not an issue because the measure is self-report. But an assessment of test–retest and internal consistency will be important to ensure that the questions are clear and nonambiguous and the items about barriers are correlated with each other. Those conditions will allow for the creation of a robust variable representing the construct *barriers*. The set of questions used to represent perceived barriers can be evaluated for face and content validity by asking experts to consider the questions "Do these questions appear to be asking about barriers to healthy beverage choices?" and "Are the full range of barriers that a student might experience, including barriers related to knowledge, attitudes, and perceptions, as well as barriers in the social and physical environment, represented in the set of questions?" Criterion validity is not possible to assess since there is no gold standard for individual-level perceptions, but construct validity would be important to assess. One would expect that the greater students' perceptions about barriers for making healthy beverage choices, the greater their consumption of SSBs or the lower their consumption of healthy beverages.

Other determinants from the social environment that the team is trying to influence are observational learning and role modeling of beverage choices from school staff, particularly teachers. Keep in mind that this assessment is not tapping students' *perceptions* of school staff behavior—those questions would be part of measures related to the individual environment; rather, it is attempting to assess behaviors of teachers while at school. In this case, the team will survey teachers about their typical beverage consumption behaviors during the school day, including what types of beverages they typically drink while at school and where students may see them consume beverages. Again, interrater reliability is not an issue because this would be a self-report instrument. However, test–retest and internal consistency, as well as content and construct validity, can be evaluated. Criterion validity would be difficult and expensive to evaluate in this example because it would require direct observation of teachers for multiple school days to establish usual beverage patterns.

Finally, to evaluate change in the availability of beverage options in the school's physical environment, the team will need to find or develop an audit tool to document what is available. An audit tool may focus on beverages available in vending machines throughout the school. In this case, interrater reliability is important to assess and would require scheduling at least two data collectors to independently complete the audit tool at the same time in the same school. If the tool, protocol, and training are clear, the two sets of data collected should be in close agreement. Test–retest reliability would involve having a data collector use the same form and protocol at two time points (often 2 weeks apart) to examine the consistency of the data collected. If consistency is low, it may indicate that the form, protocol, or training may need to be improved as the data collector saw the environment differently at the two time periods, or it may show that the environment changes over time. If the latter is the case, data collection may need to occur multiple times, and the data may need to be averaged to create a more reliable estimate of usual availability. Although face validity and content validity can be easily assessed by looking at the data collection form and related protocol, collecting criterion validity would require getting product placement data from the vending company to determine exactly what products are offered in machines over time. Construct validity would verify that there was some degree of relationship in the right direction for availability of SSBs in vending and student consumption patterns.

Where Do Teams Find Valid and Reliable Measurement Tools and Methods?

Identifying the best method or tool to assess the dependent variable (the health behavior of interest) is a crucial consideration for evaluation. Because assessing behavior is so challenging and having a valid and reliable dependent variable is so important, most teams will be better off finding an existing tool rather than trying to create their own. The Behavioral Risk Factor Surveillance System (BRFSS; CDC, n.d.-a) and the Youth Risk Behavior Surveillance System (YRBSS; CDC, n.d.-e) are excellent sources for behavioral measures. Both are conducted and organized through the CDC and are used to provide information on the prevalence of health behaviors in the U.S. population. These data allow comparisons of risk trends over time and comparisons by geographic regions and subpopulations. In addition, these data sources are used by the U.S. government to monitor progress toward achieving Healthy People and other national health objectives. Although both the BRFSS and the YRBSS were designed for the purpose of population-level health surveillance, the questions used to assess behaviors are often used in program evaluation and behavioral intervention research and also as a way to assess behavioral change, as behavioral covariates, or as a way to compare the behavior of the study population with state or national data.

The BRFSS collects state-level data on U.S. residents regarding their health-related risk behaviors, chronic health conditions, and use of preventive services; some local data are also collected. As an example, the 2019 BRFSS and its available modules included questions to assess tobacco use, alcohol consumption, marijuana consumption, PA, intake of fruits and vegetables, sodium- or salt-restriction behavior, indoor tanning, excess sun exposure, immunization, behavior related to HIV and AIDS risk, and vaccination and screening behaviors. Although the BRFSS is conducted using phone interviews, many of the questions to assess behavior have been adapted for use in written surveys and are used as a measure of health behavior for program evaluation and research projects.

Likewise, the YRBSS is a system of school-based surveys conducted with representative samples of ninth- through 12th-grade students every 2 years. The YRBSS monitors six categories of health-related behaviors that contribute to the leading causes of morbidity and mortality among youth, including behaviors that contribute to unintentional injuries and violence, sexual behaviors related to unintended pregnancy and sexually transmitted disease, alcohol and other drug use, tobacco use, unhealthy dietary behaviors, and inadequate PA. The YRBSS uses written surveys to collect these data, and the survey questions are available on the YRBSS website. In addition to these sources, the published literature and expert recommendations from specific behavioral fields can be used to identify the behavioral measures representing the state of the science.

Searching for valid and reliable measurement tools and methods to assess determinants of behavior presents additional challenges. The measurement team has three options: (a) find and use existing tools, (b) adapt existing tools to better suit their specific needs and population, or (c) create new tools. The team should start by trying to find measurement tools or methods that have already been developed and tested in a similar target population and found to have good reliability and validity. Some evidence of reliability and validity is better than no evidence, and it may not be possible to find a tool that perfectly matches the target audience and has been shown to be reliable and valid across all psychometric measures. When choosing to use an existing tool, find the most robust measure the team can afford that has been tested in a target audience as similar to the community of interest as possible.

As another option, existing tools may be adapted to better meet the needs of the specific project. For example, the team may find a set of questions tapping perceived barriers in the published literature with established reliability and validity and used in a similar population to target the behavior of interest. However, the scale misses some important barriers that are identified through formative assessment with their community. Rather than start from scratch, the team can adapt the existing scale. That adaptation should involve using the same format for asking questions and the same response options but adding or substituting questions specific to the barriers identified through formative assessment. Likewise, an observational audit tool with established reliability and validity for assessing fresh fruits and vegetables in corner stores may be identified, but important fruits and vegetables specific to the target community's food culture are missing from the audit tool. Adding or substituting new items to the existing audit, using the same format and response pattern and using the same measurement protocol will likely be more efficient and result in a more robust measurement tool than creating a new tool. Some assessment of the reliability and validity of the adapted tool should occur as part of the pilot work of the study. More specific guidelines for adapting measurement tools that have been shown to be valid and reliable in other populations are just emerging (Foti et al., 2020).

Although it may seem appealing to create survey items or measurement tools to meet the specific needs of the project, do not underestimate the difficulty of this task. It is challenging to write survey questions, design new audit tools, and develop unambiguous and complete measurement protocol (Fowler, 2014). In addition, creating new items requires evaluating their psychometric properties and creating a timeline and budget that reflect the iterative process of developing new instruments.

Choosing the best measures to use for a multicentered intervention can be especially challenging, requiring some expertise in a wide range of areas to identify the most pertinent and robust measures. Increasingly, there is a move to develop repositories of measures to be used in multilevel, transdisciplinary research. These repositories not only help research teams identify robust measures but also may help advance the field at large; more consistent use of robust measures across studies will allow for comparison of outcomes and help identify determinants that are most related to the health outcome of interest (MacLean et al., 2018). The following section provides two examples of repositories or measurement registries associated with obesity: the Accumulating Data to Optimize Obesity Treatment (ADOPT) repository and the measures registry of the National Collaborative on Childhood Obesity Research (NCCOR).

Sample Measurement Repositories Related to Obesity

The long-term vision of the ADOPT project is to work toward more effective, tailored treatments for reducing adult obesity, including both treatment and prevention approaches (MacLean et al., 2018). To achieve that vision, the project provides obesity researchers with guidance on the selection of a set of constructs (or determinants) and measures that are related to weight control. These constructs span and integrate four obesity-related domains: behavioral, biological, environmental, and psychosocial. To begin the repository, a set of constructs and related measures to be included in the repository were chosen by a team of 43 scientists who were selected for their expertise in one or more of the identified domains. Each team was asked to recommend a prioritized set of constructs to be included (based on the evidence that the construct had been consistently associated with an obesity outcome) and a set of associated measures used to assess each construct (based on the quality of the measure, including its demonstrated validity and reliability, the feasibility of using the measure in an intervention trial, and the participant burden associated with the measure). The final set of constructs and measures are included in the Grid Enabled Measurement (GEM) system, a public shared resource (https://www.gem-measures.org/). In addition, a set of articles were published to describe how the decisions were made for each domain (Lytle et al., 2018; Rosenbaum et al., 2018; Saelens et al., 2018; Sutin et al., 2018). The GEM system allows scientists to add information and study results on the existing measures and contribute newly created measures and related findings to the ADOPT database. As such, ADOPT provides a platform for growing the science and providing immediate and tangible information to inform the development of useful measurement tools specific to the field of obesity (Truong & Aronne, 2018).

The NCCOR is a partnership of the National Institutes of Health, the CDC, the U.S. Department of Agriculture, and the Robert Wood Johnson Foundation with the goal of accelerating progress in reducing childhood obesity for all children, with particular attention to high-risk populations and communities (https://www.nccor.org/). NCCOR provides a variety of resources to practitioners and researchers working in the field of childhood obesity, including a catalog of surveillance systems, a measures registry suite, a guide to methods for assessing childhood obesity, and a youth compendium for PA. The catalog of surveillance systems includes a searchable data base for diet-related, PA-related, weight-related, and geocoded or linked measures related to obesity. NCCOR also includes measurement resources specific to high-risk populations and a tool that helps teams decide whether to use existing measures, adapt measures, or develop a new measure (Foti et al., 2020).

The Measures Registry provides users with a searchable database that includes more than 200 measures and more than 1,400 supporting articles describing the psychometric properties of the tools and how they have been used in the field. The Measures Registry is populated by its users, helping to keep its content up-to-date. The Measurement Registry is organized around four domains: (a) individual diet, (b) individual PA, (c) food environment, and (d) PA environment. Users begin by choosing a domain and measurement type (e.g., GIS, 24-hour recall, food frequency, electronic monitor, environmental observation, questionnaire, record or log). They can also narrow their search by the age group of interest and context of interest (metro/urban or small town/rural environment). Once the domain of interest and the other descriptors are identified, a list of potentially useful measurement tools is displayed. For each tool in the registry, the relevant citation for the published source of the tool is included, along with an abstract, information on how the measurement tool was used in the original study, and available information on the reliability and validity of the tool. In most cases the full text of the article and the assessment instrument are also available. Included in the Measures Registry suite are a set of user's guides for each of the four domains, learning modules that provide overviews of key measurement concepts for users newer to research and evaluation, a guide to the registry for those preparing grant applications, and a guide to the registry for educators.

ADOPT and NCCOR are two examples of measurement repositories that are beginning to be developed by specific content areas. Many others are available for other behavioral content areas and may provide important sources of recommended measurement tools. The RAND Online Measure Repository provides an online searchable database containing measures related to psychological health (RAND Corporation, n.d.). The PhenX Toolkit (https://www.phenxtoolkit.org/) provides recommended data collection protocols for conducting biomedical research funded by the National Human Genome Research Institute and includes measures and measurement protocol across a large number of domains, including alcohol, tobacco, and other substance use; oral health; and psychosocial and social environments.

Examining How Well the Conceptual Model Worked: Mediation and Moderation Analysis

The primary focus of the evaluation is to answer the question "Was the intervention effective in changing the behavior targeted?" Although examining the effectiveness of the intervention is crucial, it explains little about the mechanisms through which the intervention worked or groups that may have responded differentially to the intervention. The conceptual model that was developed as part of the Plan Phase suggests that change in behavior will occur by making a positive impact on the determinants that are addressed through the intervention. In other words, change in determinants is expected to *mediate* the relationship between the intervention and the behavioral outcome. The conceptual model also includes suggestions of characteristics of the sample that may differentially influence or *moderate* the relationships of constructs within the conceptual model.

Figure 6.2 shows pictures of the relationships being tested through mediation and moderation analysis. *Mediation analysis* examines the extent to which a proposed mediator directly and indirectly influences the dependent variable. Full mediation occurs when all of the variance in the dependent variable can be explained by change in the mediator; partial mediation occurs when only some of the variance in the dependent variable can be directly attributed to the mediator. As an example, assume that the independent variable represents the treatment condition (control or intervention group), the dependent variable is the behavior that is being targeted, and the mediator in question represents a determinant of the behavior—for example, participant's motivation to change. A full mediation model would suggest that all the impact of the intervention occurred by increasing individuals' motivation to change, while the partial mediation model would suggest that although some of the variance in behavior change can be attributed to a change in motivation, there is additional variance in behavior change that is attributed to some other factor or factors related to the treatment condition. Conceptual models produced for an MLI will predict partial mediation as determinants from multiple environmental levels will be expected to contribute to the change in behavior. The expected effect from each level or determinant is typically not estimated a priori. Rather, synergy is expected between levels and the independent and combined contributions of determinants toward effecting behavior change are determined post hoc (Zyphur et al., 2019).

FIGURE 6.2. Mediation and Moderation

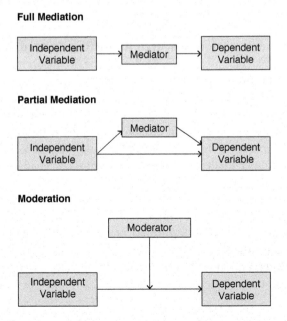

In addition, the conceptual model should include a list of possible moderators. In behavioral research, a *moderator* is some characteristic of the sample that is identified as possibly influencing the relationship between the independent variable and the dependent variable. Moderators should be identified a priori as the conceptual model is being designed based on what other research has shown or common sense. Moderators identified after data are collected and analyzed should be considered exploratory analysis; searching for moderators post hoc (after the results are known) may lead to Type I error rate inflation.

Example of Examining Mediators and Moderators Through the Conceptual Model: Healthy Teens, Healthy Planet

As an example of both mediation and moderation, the conceptual model that was built in the Plan Phase for Healthy Teens, Healthy Planet (see Chapter 3) shows that the team believes that the intervention will result in a change in adolescent consumption of SSB through eight specific determinants at three environmental levels: At the individual level, through positive change in students' perceived control, perceived barriers, and knowledge; at the social level, through positive change in role modeling, descriptive norms, and social reinforcement; and at the physical level, through changes in the availability of beverage choices at school and the relative cost (accessibility) of beverages available at school (Figure 6.3). The conceptual model posits that these eight determinants will mediate the relationship between the independent variable signifying the treatment condition and adolescent SSB consumption. In designing the intervention, the team cannot say which determinant will have the strongest effect on changing behavior, but as part of data analysis, the team will be able to quantifiably estimate the impact of the total intervention as well as the impact of each mediator on the variance in behavior change. As for potential moderators, the team hypothesized that the intervention may be differentially received by urban compared with suburban schools, by size of school enrollment, and by student gender. Moderation analysis allows the team to examine whether those assumptions were correct.

Examples of Intervention Research Reporting on Mediators and Moderators

In this section, I provide two examples of how examining mediators and moderators has added to the understanding of how, and for whom, interventions work. The Smart Moms study (Nezami et al., 2020) examined the extent to which a family-based intervention positively influenced the determinants targeted in the intervention through a mediation analysis; the Women's Lifestyle PA program examined moderators of treatment impact on change in PA behavior (Schoeny et al., 2017).

The Smart Moms intervention was a 6-month, maternal-targeted intervention to reduce SSB intake and fruit juice consumption in children aged 3 to 5 years. After baseline data collection, 51 mother–child dyads were randomly assigned to receive the Smart Moms intervention or to a waitlist control group. Those in the intervention group participated in one face-to-face group session and a mobile-optimized website that included 12 weekly lessons followed by

FIGURE 6.3. Example Mediators and Moderators: The Healthy Teens/Healthy Planet Intervention to Reduce the Intake of Sugar-Sweetened Beverages (SSBs)

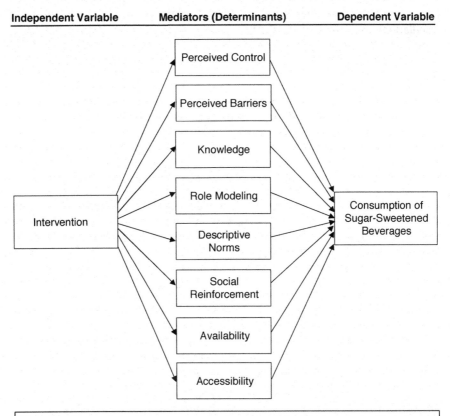

Potential Moderators: Urban versus suburban school district; size of school/enrollment; gender

six biweekly lessons. The intervention was designed to positively influence the following determinants across all three environmental levels: self-efficacy and outcome expectations (individual environment); maternal SSB and juice consumption, the structure of family meals, the use of food as rewards, parental limiting of foods (100% fruit juice and SSBs), and parental concern about the child's diet (social environment); and limiting foods (fruits and vegetables and fruit juice) available in the home (physical environment). The outcome evaluation for the study showed that after the 6-month intervention, children in the Smart Moms intervention group had a significant reduction in SSB and juice intake compared with children in the control group (Nezami et al., 2018).

The goal of the mediation study (Nezami et al., 2020) was to examine whether the intervention positively influenced these 10 determinants in the first 3 months of the study and, subsequently, if the determinants operated as mediators of the effect of the intervention on changes in child SSB and juice consumption measured at 6 months. The results suggested that at 3 months, mothers in the Smart Moms group compared with mothers in the waitlist control group had a statistically significant change in four of the 10 determinants: a decrease in their own

SSB or juice intake, an increase in limit setting for 100% fruit juice, an increase in the availability of fruits and vegetables in the home, and a decrease in parental concern about child's diet. Those four variables were then tested in a multiple mediation model to examine the direct and indirect effects of the change in each of those determinants on the primary outcome (child's SSB and juice intake at 6 months). The only determinant found to be a significant mediator was maternal beverage consumption at 3 months, suggesting that the reduction in mothers' caloric beverage intake at 3 months explained a statistically significant amount of the variance in child's beverage intake at 6 months.

The results from this mediation analysis suggest that future interventions targeting children's intake of SSB should include a strong component to address mothers' behavior. Although the findings did not show that other targeted determinants were related to the primary outcome, that does not mean they should be ignored in future interventions. The strong findings around mothers' behavior likely reflect not only role-modeling but also other aspects of the individual, social, and physical environment that changed as a result of the intervention but were not picked up by the measurement tools. In addition, it may be that the intervention strategies designed to have an impact on the determinants were not strong enough, and future iterations of the intervention need to focus on improving them. These important insights would have been missed without a mediation analysis.

The goal of the Women's Lifestyle PA program was to evaluate the effectiveness of an intervention to increase adherence to lifestyle PA in midlife (ages 40–65) African American women (Wilbur et al., 2016). The intervention was designed to compare the effectiveness of a standard treatment using group meetings with the addition of follow-up calls with a nurse facilitator using motivational interviewing or follow-up automated phone calls. The sample included 284 women randomized to one of three treatment groups: (a) six group meetings that focused on addressing barriers and correcting misinformation about PA through a video and group discussions, (b) six group meetings plus 11 calls with a nurse facilitator using motivational interviewing to help participants explore and resolve their ambivalence about increasing activity levels, and (c) six group meetings plus 11 automated telephone calls with motivational problem-solving tips. Adherence to PA at baseline, 24 weeks, and 48 weeks was assessed by self-report PA questionnaires, accelerometry, and by an aerobic fitness test. The analysis conducted to evaluate the effectiveness of the intervention found that all three conditions significantly improved women's adherence to PA overtime but that there were no significant differences between conditions (Wilbur et al., 2016).

Additional analyses were conducted to examine potential moderators of the intervention effect, specifically potential barriers experienced by these women, including demographic factors (number of children in the household, employment status, and material hardship), physical health (perceptions of general health, global pain, and body mass index), psychological health (depression), perceived barriers to PA, social support for PA from family and friends, and neighborhood factors (perceived walkability of the neighborhood and rates of aggravated assaults/battery as obtained from police departments; Schoeny et al., 2017). The moderators to be examined were specified a priori (before any analyses were conducted) and selected on the basis of existing evidence that these barriers may interfere with one's ability to be physically active and may be expected to affect the relationship between the intervention being evaluated and PA as an outcome. Moderation was examined using a three-way interaction analysis looking at Barriers × Condition × Time.

Focusing only on the analysis done using accelerometer data as the measure of PA, the investigators found significant interactions between study condition and PA levels for five of the barriers: material hardship, general health, depression, neighborhood assault rate, and perceived barriers to physical activity. Baseline depression emerged as the strongest moderator of treatment effects. For those participants with higher levels of baseline depression, those randomized to either group with supplemental calls improved their PA as measured in number of steps over and above those just attending the group sessions. Although the mechanism of the additional phone calls is not clear, it may be that the phone calls helped boost self-efficacy or added important problem-solving skills for those experiencing higher levels of barriers (Schoeny et al., 2017). These results add to what was learned from the study because it showed that five moderators were found, including some at the individual and neighborhood levels. Although future iterations of this intervention will not be able to have a direct impact on these moderators, knowing that these conditions will affect how the intervention is received by participants is crucial. It may suggest that the intervention needs to build in a social support component to help participants cope with the challenges of their life situation, or it may suggest that a different type of intervention may be more effective for participants with these challenges. Although

INSIGHTS FOR INTERVENTIONISTS: WHAT DO WE LEARN ABOUT HOW INTERVENTIONS WORK THROUGH MEDIATION AND MODERATION?

There is much to be gained by understanding how interventions work through mediation and moderation analysis. When mediation analysis shows that behavioral determinants were not affected by the intervention, as interventionists, we learn that our intervention strategies need to be stronger. When mediation analysis shows that determinants were changed by the intervention but did not lead to change in behavior, we learn that the intervention efforts may need to focus on change in other determinants. When we learn that characteristics of the individual, social, or physical environment expressed as moderators affect how interventions work, we learn that we may need to design or adapt interventions for groups with different characteristics. Without that information, our ability to make meaningful strides in designing interventions that work will be stymied.

an intervention focusing on increasing PA will not be prepared to deal with the larger social issues that were found to be important, documenting and communicating about those disparities is important public health work.

Design and Analysis Issues for Group- or Cluster-Randomized Trials

MLIs are often evaluated as group- or cluster-randomized trials. Group- or cluster-randomized trials evaluate interventions operating at the group level that observe individual members of those groups to assess the effects of the intervention (Murray, 1998; Murray et al., 2010). Interventions attempting to change the walkability of neighborhoods, reduce vaping at a worksite, or reduce students' SSB consumption at school are all interventions implemented at the group or organizational level, but their effectiveness is based on measurements taken from individuals within those groups or organizations. For example, although an intervention may work to create a more walkable neighborhood environment by adding sidewalks and bike paths, activity patterns of individuals within those neighborhoods are measured to assess the impact of the intervention.

Group- or cluster-randomized trials bring some unique challenges for those planning the evaluation. I have learned practical lessons about the evaluation of MLIs through my decades of experience as the behavioral scientist working with biostatisticians and epidemiologists to design and evaluate MLI trials. In this section, I highlight some of the issues that the interventionist or behavior scientist on a team should understand at a conceptual level but rely on the expertise of other team members to manage—specifically, sample size considerations, randomizing by blocking, accounting for individuals nested in groups, the potential for contamination in group- or cluster-randomized trials, recruiting for such trials, and examining the independent and synergistic effects of intervention components.

Sample Size Considerations

Estimating sample size is a topic beyond the scope of this volume, but it is important to know that there are sample size considerations unique to group- or cluster-randomized trials. In these types of trials, groups are assigned to a treatment condition. Therefore, the study is powered on the number of groups to be randomized, not the number of people within each group. For example, a study that randomizes eight churches to a control or intervention condition and measures 250 parishioners from each church has a sample size of eight, not 2,000. Designing MLIs that have adequate power to detect intervention effects requires a sufficient number of group-level units. Having too few groups decreases the power of the study and increases the chance of a Type II error, suggesting that the intervention was not successful when it was. On the other hand, engaging more groups than are needed for a study can tie up resources that could be used toward strengthening the intervention (Murray et al., 2007). Ignoring groups in the analysis can result in an inflated the Type I error rate, suggesting that the intervention was a success when it was not. Describing how one calculates the required sample size for a group- or cluster-randomized trials is beyond the scope of this book, but many excellent sources exist. Practitioners are particularly directed to *Design and Analysis of Group-Randomized Trials* (Murray, 1998), *Power Analysis of Trials With Multilevel Data* (Moerbeek & Teerenstra, 2016), and a National Institutes of Health website designed to provide more information on group- and cluster-randomized trials (https://researchmethodsresources. nih.gov/).

Randomizing by Blocking

Another issue with randomizing groups rather than individuals is that it is difficult for simple randomization to evenly distribute potential sources of confounding. In intervention trials that randomize individuals to condition, the sample sizes required are usually large enough that randomization will work fairly well to distribute potential confounders equally between treatment groups. However, group- or cluster-randomized trials engage a smaller number of units, making it more difficult to rely on simple randomization. To help increase the potential that randomization will result in equivalent groups, group- or cluster-randomized trials often use block randomization or stratification; the units to be randomized are grouped by some characteristics, and randomization occurs within the block. As an example, in the TEENS study (described in Chapters 4 and 5), before randomization, the 16 TEENS schools were matched based on the proportion of seventh graders within a school expected to receive the curriculum (based on course requirements at each school), the proportion of seventh graders qualifying for free and reduced lunch in each school, and the size of the school (Murray et al., 2007). One school was randomly assigned to a condition from each pair. This increased the chance that the schools in the control and intervention conditions would have approximately the same proportion of seventh-grade students expected to receive the condition and an equal distribution of students qualifying for free and reduced lunch; it also ensured that the four smallest schools would be distributed between the control and intervention conditions (Janega et al., 2004a). Although TEENS used pair-matching in randomizing units to condition (assigning one school from each pair to condition at a time), current thought is that randomly assigning two groups to each condition from each stratum is preferable to reduce the chances of a Type I error (Donner et al., 2007).

Individuals Nested Within Groups: Accounting for Intraclass Correlation

In group- or cluster-randomized trials, groups represent both the unit of randomization and analysis, but measures are taken from individuals within those groups to assess the effectiveness of the intervention. Individuals who are measured are "nested" within the group and share some physical, social, geographic, or other commonalities with others in the group. For example, imagine an intervention to reduce the risk factors for prediabetes in adults. The intervention will be offered to residents of low-income housing units, and housing units will be randomized to treatment condition. Residents from each housing unit will likely have some things in common. For example, they share neighborhood characteristics such as the availability of fresh produce or walking paths in proximity to where they live. They share many elements of their social environments because behavioral patterns of those living in the housing units will be observable, providing vicarious learning and creating social norms. In addition, housing units may include relatives that share both genetic and behavioral traits. Common attributes shared by the group mean that the measures taken at the individual level are not truly independent. Independence is a critical assumption for statistics requiring that the value of one observation does not influence or affect the value of other observations (Murray et al., 2007). A violation of that assumption will increase the risk of a Type I error rate.

A statistical adjustment to correct for the "sameness" that exists between individuals within a group must occur. The sameness is referred to as the intraclass correlation coefficient (ICC) and reflects an extra component of variance that is seen in the dependent variable because individuals are nested within the group randomized to condition. This extra variation will increase the variation of any group-level statistic beyond what would be expected if individuals, rather than groups, were randomized to condition. If the ICC is not accounted for analytically, the Type I error rate can be badly inflated. Reflecting the ICC in the analysis helps correct for these nonindependent measures. ICC estimates can be obtained from published studies reporting similar outcomes, with a similar population, using a similar unit of randomization and study design and analytic strategy (Blitstein et al., 2005; Murray et al., 2007). As examples, three papers from the TEENS study were published to provide ICC estimates for a variety of behavioral endpoints measured in adolescents (Janega et al., 2004a, 2004b; Murray et al., 2001).

As a side note, ICCs may be important to consider even when individuals are randomized to condition. When individuals are recruited from existing groups the correlation between individuals still exist and must be accounted for analytically. As an example, in the CHOICES study, young adults were recruited from three community colleges but randomized as individuals to either the control or intervention arm of the study (Lytle, Moe, et al., 2014; Lytle et al., 2017). In CHOICES, individual students were randomized from within blocks defined by college, weight status, and gender. Those factors were included in the analysis as covariates to improve the power for the analysis of the intervention effect.

The Potential for Contamination in Group- or Cluster-Randomized Trials

Contamination occurs when an individual or group randomized to the control condition is exposed to some element of the intervention. Imagine, for example, a clinic-based intervention to promote colorectal screening with randomization occurring at the level of provider. Some providers in the clinic are trained to deliver the intervention protocol (which involves delivering a specific health message to patients about screening), while other clinicians are to continue to deliver usual care. The study is evaluated by comparing patient screening rates between physicians in the control versus intervention conditions. A study design that involves randomizing providers within a clinic risks contamination from at least two sources: (a) providers within a clinic may talk with each other and cue the importance of reminding patients about screening and (b) patients may not always see the same provider. If patients of providers randomized to the control condition are exposed to the messages about screening, the control condition is contaminated. To make sure the study is designed to avoid the potential for contamination requires that randomization to a condition occurs at the highest level of change. In this case, contamination would be eliminated by randomizing clinics to condition, as long as physicians did not work across clinics.

Recruiting for Group- or Cluster-Randomized Trials
In group- or cluster-randomized trials, the recruitment process begins with recruiting groups to be involved in the study, not individuals. Recruiting groups requires involving community stakeholders in the plans and an appreciation for the amount of time it may take to recruit the required sample. As an example, in the TEENS study, we wanted to target the intervention to a lower income population; therefore, we restricted our recruitment to schools where at least 20% of the student population was eligible for free or reduced lunches (Lytle et al., 2004). Our recruitment process began with identifying schools that met this criterion within a 45-minute drive of the university. Distance was an important consideration because of the time and expense involved for both measurement and intervention staff to visit schools. We identified 33 schools across 14 school districts in the metro area of Minneapolis and St. Paul that met this criterion. Once those schools were identified, we contacted the school superintendent from each district to have an initial conversation regarding their level of interest in the project. If they expressed interest, we met with principals and teachers from the schools to talk about the project. This step typically involved scheduling face-to-face meetings at the school, where our team made a brief presentation about the topic and engaged with school stakeholders to get their thoughts about the project. Getting support from school staff, in addition to the support from school administration, took additional time and meetings. Although administrative support was necessary, the success of the intervention rested on the support and cooperation of teachers and school food service staff who would be more closely involved in implementing it.

The process of recruiting schools took approximately 3 months to complete. Twenty schools were interested in participating; one school was used for the pilot phase, and three other schools were excluded due to scheduling conflicts. Once the schools were recruited, we approached the task of recruiting students within each school to participate in TEENS measurements. Sample size calculations to test our primary hypotheses were based on fruit, vegetable, and fat intake data from prior school-based studies (and adjusted with estimates of ICC for each outcome). These calculations indicated that with 16 schools and at least 30 students measured per school, the study had 80% power to detect differences of 1.1 serving of fruits and vegetables and a 1.9% difference in energy from total fat between treatment groups (Lytle et al., 2004). The 16 schools were randomized (using block randomization) after baseline data collection to control or intervention conditions and included more than 3,500 students. On the basis of sample size calculations, we would have been adequately powered to test our primary hypotheses by collecting data on 480 students (30 students at 16 schools), but it was simpler logistically to recruit all of the students in the appropriate grade level and ensure that enough students were exposed to the classroom curriculum component. The larger sample size also allowed us to do many secondary and exploratory analyses at the individual level.

Examining the Independent and Synergistic Effects of Intervention Components on Behavior Change

Another important study design issue related to MLIs is the ability to examine independent and synergistic effects of intervention components. Consider the Healthy Teens, Healthy Planet example, the school-based intervention to reduce adolescent SSB consumption. The intervention has three components: a curriculum, a social media campaign, and policy and practice approaches. To evaluate the effectiveness of the intervention as a whole, there are two comparison groups, or factors, to be tested: schools that receive the intervention and schools that do not receive the intervention. The hypothesis is as follows: Youth from schools that are randomized to receive the intervention consume fewer servings of SSBs compared with youth attending schools who do not receive the intervention.

To test this hypothesis, schools are randomized to condition, making schools the unit of randomization and analysis. Consumption of SSBs is estimated using a validated beverage screener to be completed by a sample of students in each school. Sample size is calculated using an estimate of the average mean intake and variance estimates for SSB consumption in youth. For this example, assume that sample size calculations determined that a total of 16 schools with at least 30 students per school were needed to have 80% power to estimate a 0.5 serving size difference in SSB consumption with the significance level set at 0.05. After baseline data collection, the 16 schools would be matched on a few relevant characteristics such as the proportion of students receiving free or reduced meals and a blocked or stratified randomization used to assign schools to condition.

If the goal was to examine the independent or synergistic effects of the three components, the research question would be: "What intervention components are most effective in reducing SSB in adolescents?" To answer this question, a comparison of eight factors would be necessary based on the presence or absence of three components (represented factorially as 2^3 or $2 \times 2 \times 2$). The eight factors would be as follows:

- control condition
- curriculum only
- social media campaign only
- school-wide policy and practices only

- curriculum plus social media campaign
- curriculum plus school-wide policy and practices
- social media campaign plus school-wide policy and practices
- curriculum plus social media campaign plus school-wide policy and practices

This full factorial design would be able to test the impact of each separate component and also evaluate all possible combinations of components. Randomization into condition using block randomization would still be required, and the number of schools needed to have the power to answer these questions would be very large, possibly as many as 64 schools (eight schools per each of eight conditions). The study would not likely be affordable (Cleary et al., 2012; Murray et al., 2010).

It is possible to do a simpler design when specific hypotheses are tested. For example, the group might be interested in how the school-wide policy and practice component influences SSBs consumption as compared with an intervention that includes all three components. In that case, the study could be designed to randomize schools to one of three conditions: (a) control, (b) school-wide policy and practices component, and (c) the intervention as a whole, including all three components, and may require only 24 schools (eight schools per three conditions). By identifying the specific combination of intervention components to evaluate for synergy, the number of units required to recruit is diminished providing a more cost-effective approach (Cleary et al., 2012; Murray et al., 2010).

Examining Change and Maintenance of Change

It is important to consider the timing and number of measurement points to plan for the study. For pilot work and studies with limited resources, two measurement periods (baseline and postintervention) are often used. A post-only option is also acceptable, but having a baseline measure as a way to confirm comparability of groups is highly desirable. Beyond those two essential measurement periods, additional ones should be considered as a way to evaluate the patterns and the maintenance of change.

Practically, the number of measurement points to include in the study design is both a resource and time issue. More measurement periods will require additional staff time to collect and clean data and track participants. More measurement periods place additional burden on participants and typically mean higher attrition rates, exacerbating concerns about the generalizability of findings. In addition, more measurements could focus more attention on the outcomes of interest to the study, increasing both the control and intervention groups' sensitivity to the importance of these outcomes and thus creating bias. More measurement periods add to the financial needs related to offering incentives to participants as well as travel expenses.

The number of measurement periods to plan for is a conceptual issue as well. It may be that for some behaviors, showing effective change in the short term will be a significant and important finding. Newly developed interventions and interventions targeting health behaviors that are intermittent rather than daily (e.g., health screening, vaccination, dental checkups) may appropriately evaluate their effectiveness by using a simple pre–post measurement schedule. However, for interventions that focus on behaviors that occur daily, such as eating, physical activity, oral hygiene, or avoiding cigarettes, assessing the maintenance of the behavior may be as important as assessing initial change. If maintenance of change is an important question for the study, measurement periods will be needed before the intervention, immediately after the intervention, and at one or more follow-up periods.

The optimal outcome for behavior change interventions focusing on daily behaviors is sustained behavior change rather than temporary change. Positive impact on physiological or biological outcomes requires behavior changes that persist over time. However, there is some evidence to suggest that the processes and challenges related to initial behavior change differ from the processes and challenges of maintaining behavior change. Many interventions that are effective in creating initial behavior change may not result in long-term change. As an example, in the field of adult weight loss interventions, it is well documented that interventions can be effective in helping people lose weight and maintain that weight loss for about 3 months, after which, the majority of individuals relapse and begin regaining weight (Weiss et al., 2007). Therefore, consideration of the number and timing of measurement points requires a consideration of potential relapse patterns for the behavior of interest.

Relapse prevention is a health behavior theory that addresses the challenges in sustaining behavior change and avoiding relapse, particularly for addictive and indulgent behaviors such as smoking, drinking, drug use, and overeating (Marlatt & Donovan, 2005; Marlatt & Gordon, 1985). Marlatt's work shows a consistent and comparable relapse effect that occurs after approximately 3 months of initial behavior change in these behaviors and considers the unique challenges of maintaining behavior change.

Relapse prevention focuses on helping individuals avoid high-risk situations, build self-efficacy for the healthy behavior, change outcome expectancies,

RELAPSE PREVENTION: CHALLENGES ASSOCIATED WITH MAINTAINING A BEHAVIOR CHANGE

- High-risk situations that will inevitably occur and tempt the individual to revert to their previous behavioral choices
- Low self-efficacy for one's ability to resist the urge to engage in the unhealthy behavior
- The expected value or outcome expectancy about the pleasure to be experienced from the unhealthy behavior
- Guilt that results from a slip or lapse and precipitates lack of self-control

and learn that a slip in behavior is a learning opportunity rather than a failure. Relapse prevention suggests that, particularly for addictive or indulgent behaviors, measuring behavior 3 months after the end of the intervention period would provide important information related to sustained change.

Likewise, for interventions targeting organizational or policy change, it is obvious that the goal is permanent change, or institutionalization, of those changes. As interventionists, we would like the new program that is developed, implemented, and found effective in improving the health of a community to be fully adopted and continued even after the implementation and evaluation steps are complete. Likewise, to be effective, new policies and practices established as a result of the intervention need to become accepted as the new norm, supported, and held up over time across a variety of administrators, policy makers, and stakeholders. The institutionalization of programs requires organizational commitment, however, and this includes incorporating the program into the organization's mission, standard operations, and budget (Bracht, 1990). Too often programs are dropped or substantially diluted after the intervention trial is complete. Likewise, policies and practices can be dropped or diluted when new policy makers are in charge or when the problem stream changes (Kingdon, 2011). Changes that involved a substantial change to the physical space are likely to be more permanent (e.g., building a walking path around the perimeter of a worksite's campus), but it is easy to imagine that policy and practice changes that affect the individual or social environment (e.g., offering employee wellness classes, providing behavioral incentives) may be abandoned if a new administration takes over or if substantial change in the larger environment occurs. If a goal of an intervention is the institutionalization of organizational or policy change, measuring the environmental outcomes related to those changes should be measured over time and not just at the end of the active intervention phase.

Even though the importance of measuring sustained change is intuitive, there is limited research showing the long-term effects of interventions on either individuals or system-level intervention targets. The paucity of research in this area is largely due to limited resources and difficulties in tracking individuals, as well as the challenges of conducting assessments of programs, practices, and policies in organizations, over time. In addition, timing for funding streams often does not match with this goal. Too much time may lapse between the end of an intervention trial and when funding is secured to evaluate the sustained impact of the intervention on individuals or institutions; by the time funding is obtained, individuals can no longer be located, and institutions may have lost their interest in participating in research. The paucity of research on the long-term impact of MLIs to promote population health may also reflect a health research focus with strong roots in medicine and clinical practice where the intervention is a drug or medical procedure that "cures" the individual, reducing the perceived need for follow-up.

For MLIs designed to promote population health, the goal is to design interventions that are effective in creating and sustaining behavior change of individuals by positively influencing the environments that influence their behaviors.

Therefore, intervention research should support the rigorous testing of interventions for their effectiveness as well as evaluations of the long-term impact of the intervention on the behaviors of individuals and the environments that are changed by the interventions.

There are limited examples of MLI research that have examined an intervention's impact on effectiveness as well as the sustainability of change at the individual and environmental levels. The CATCH school-based MLI to reduce cardiovascular risk in elementary school children (described in some detail in Chapter 1, this volume), stands as an exception (Luepker et al., 1996). Following the evaluation of the intervention in 96 schools across four sites, two additional grants were awarded as follow-up studies to CATCH: the CATCH Tracking study (Nader et al., 1999) and the CATCH Institutionalization study (Parcel et al., 2003).

The purpose of the CATCH Tracking study was to evaluate the persistence of intervention effects on the dietary and physical activity behaviors of the CATCH cohort seen at the end of the school-based intervention. The CATCH Tracking study followed the original cohort of students through the eighth grade, 3 years after their exposure to the CATCH intervention in Grades 3 through 5. We were able to track 3,714 (73%) of the initial cohort of 5,106 students from ethnically diverse backgrounds in California, Louisiana, Minnesota, and Texas to the end of their eighth-grade year and assessed diet (using 24-hour recalls in Grade 8 and a food checklist for Grades 7 and 8), a self-administered physical activity checklist (Grades 6–8), a health behavior survey assessing psychosocial factors including knowledge, perceived social support, and intentions for eating healthy foods (Grades 6–8), and physiological variables, including blood samples, height, weight, skinfold thickness, and blood pressure (Grade 8). The results of the tracking study showed that students who were exposed to CATCH reported significantly lower intake of total fat and significantly more minutes of daily vigorous activity compared with control students 3 years after their last exposure to the CATCH intervention. Likewise, differences between treatment groups for dietary knowledge and intent were maintained through eighth grade. As with the original CATCH intervention study, no statistically significant differences were seen in physiological outcomes between conditions (Nader et al., 1999).

The CATCH Institutionalization study (also known as CATCH-ON) was an observational study conducted 5 years after the end of the main CATCH intervention trial and designed to examine the extent of institutionalization in both intervention and control schools participating in CATCH. At the end of the CATCH main trial, the 40 control schools were provided with materials necessary to implement the CATCH program and in-service training. For this study, 20 former CATCH control schools were randomly selected to compare their implementation of CATCH with how CATCH was being implemented in the original intervention schools ($n = 56$). In addition, 12 new schools were recruited with no prior exposure to CATCH to serve as a measure of secular trends in school-based cardiovascular health promotion programs (Parcel et al., 2003). School-level intervention activities that were assessed included (a) the macronutrient content of school lunch menus, (b) the amount and type of physical education classes held in schools, and (c) health instruction practices in the classroom. In addition, an institutionalization score was developed combining these three metrics. Results suggested that 50% of the menus from former CATCH schools met the recommended guidelines for fat, compared with 10% of the menus from former control schools and 17% of the menus from unexposed schools ($p < .005$). Former CATCH intervention schools spent more time teaching CATCH heath education lessons and taught more lessons than CATCH control schools, and the overall implementation score was highest in CATCH intervention schools compared with former control schools ($p < .001$). No differences were seen with regard to the physical education goals between conditions (Hoelscher et al., 2004). Training appeared to have the largest impact on the maintenance of CATCH programs.

As part of CATCH-ON, we also conducted key informant interviews with 199 school staff, including school food service, physical education teachers, classroom teachers, and administrators at the four CATCH-ON field centers. The interviews sought to hear perspectives on the degree of CATCH program implementation, the key people in each school promoting CATCH, and the conditions that facilitated or impeded the institutionalization of CATCH activities. Implementation was mixed across components, schools, and sites. The primary barriers to implementation included competing priorities from other issues; the lack of a mechanism for continued training of school staff; and lack of sufficient funds for materials, equipment, and supporting the availability of lower fat vendor products (Lytle et al., 2003). Results from this study suggest that changes to the school environment to support healthful behaviors can be maintained over time and that finding ways to continue staff training is an important factor in achieving institutionalization of these programs.

CATCH-ON was important work because it helped evaluate the feasibility of continuing intervention activities with existing community resources and the level of relevance of the intervention to the schools. CATCH helped to answer the following important questions related to dissemination and institutionalization:

- Did schools that were involved in CATCH value the activities and outcomes of CATCH enough to continue to support them outside of a funded research trial?

- What does it take for a community to sustain programs and policies that they value?

- How do evaluated interventions change as they are disseminated?

These questions are part of the work that is done in implementation research and implementation science. *Implementation research* is the study of the processes and factors associated with successful integration of evidence-based interventions within a particular setting, whereas *implementation science* refers to the development and application of common principles, models, and designs to study and promote the uptake of evidence-based practices and policies

(Brownson et al., 2015). Implementation science is discussed in more detail in Chapter 7 of this volume.

Finalizing Evaluation Plans

As the evaluation plans are finalized, it is important to document all decisions through a written evaluation protocol or manual of operating procedures.

Details included in the protocol will be needed to describe the methods and analytic approaches of the study in published articles and reports. Including the copies of all the forms used, as well as documentation of the sources of measurement tools and survey items, will be invaluable when revisions and adaptions of the intervention are planned. In addition, finding good measurement tools is challenging, and colleagues will frequently ask for a copy of the measurement tools, their sources, and related psychometric properties. To be able to retrieve those details from one document or file saves a great deal of time. Most important, the measurement protocol, like the intervention protocol, should provide the level of detail to allow others to replicate the study and provides the transparency needed to help advance the science.

DETAILS TO INCLUDE IN THE EVALUATION PROTOCOL

- A copy of the original grant or program proposal

- The specific aims of the intervention and the hypotheses being tested, including the primary hypotheses as well as prespecified secondary outcomes and exploratory hypotheses

- A description of the assumptions used to calculate sample size, including variance estimates and other parameter estimates

- A timeline for intervention and measurement activities

- Plans for study recruitment and retention, including tools used for recruitment

- Detailed analytic models, including covariates

- Copies of all measurement protocols, including data collection procedures, forms, surveys, and audit tools

- Details of psychometric testing of measurement tools

- Documentation of the source of each measurement tool and the source of each question used in surveys

- Evaluation training materials, including details on certifying data collectors

- Copies of all documents related to the protection of human subjects

- The final CONSORT diagram and checklist to be included at the end of the study

STEP 12: PREPARE FOR THE NEXT ITERATION OR DISSEMINATION OF THE INTERVENTION

The final step in the intervention design process is to revise the intervention based on lessons learned and prepare for the next iteration or dissemination of the intervention. I distinguish this step in the design process from adapting an evidence-based intervention (discussed in Chapter 7, this volume) by seeing this step occurring with the original team that created the intervention as a way to improve and build on their own work.

As the intervention is occurring and process data are reviewed, the team will likely see some elements of the intervention that are going well but also elements that could be improved in a future iteration. As the intervention finishes and all process and outcome data are available, additional insights for ways to improve the intervention will emerge. Analysis for the primary outcome will show how effective the intervention was, and the results of the mediation and moderation analysis will provide essential information on how the intervention worked to change determinants and whether there were groups that responded to the intervention differentially.

In some cases, intervention teams will continue to work to refine a specific intervention approach and conduct many experiments altering elements of the same intervention or testing the intervention in new settings or using new technology. In other cases, intervention teams will turn to other behavior change areas or other population groups for their next project. Even in those cases, the experience gleaned from each intervention designed and tested is invaluable. Each intervention tested provides an opportunity to see how well an intervention strategy works to change a determinant; lessons learned about effective intervention strategies may translate into different behavior change interventions in which the same determinants are important. Each intervention tested provides an opportunity to see how elements of the intervention work in the community and insight into the feasibility of intervention activities including the time, skills, and resources needed to deliver the intervention as designed. Each intervention trial provides experience with data collection that is often generalizable to other studies. Most importantly, working with an engaged community stakeholder group in designing an intervention builds relationships and trust that will provide the important foundation for working together to improve the health of community.

Several things can be done to maximize what can be learned from an intervention. First, the creation of both an intervention and measurement manual of procedures is an essential task. Important details about why certain decisions were made, how a particular intervention strategy was designed, timing for intervention and evaluation activities, and procedures used to recruit and retain participants are easily forgotten by the end of a multiyear intervention trial. These documents also provide the transparency needed as other investigators adopt the intervention to meet the needs of their population.

Second, it is important to share the results of the intervention study with community stakeholders. Their perspectives on why something did not work out as planned and their thoughts about how elements of the intervention can be improved will be invaluable. If possible, conducting formative evaluation from those community stakeholders who were involved in delivering the intervention as well as recipients of the intervention may provide qualitative and quantitative information that will be helpful in explaining why the intervention worked—or why it didn't—how it worked, and for whom. Formative assessment with those who dropped out of the program before completion will be useful in highlighting barriers to participation.

Finally, dedicating time for the team to reflect on what was learned from the experience is important. Planning a retreat or dedicating blocks of time to discuss what was learned and to use that knowledge to sketch out the next iteration of the intervention is essential. Too often, intervention teams are busy beginning the next intervention study before the previous one is finished. In some cases, interventions that were ineffective may be abandoned without the team fully digesting what happened. In other cases, even promising interventions may end up on the shelf because of other priorities, resulting in only a single published manuscript. Data that have been carefully collected are left in data files with no one to do analyses, leaving many clues for how to improve intervention efforts undisclosed.

In many cases, lack of funding causes this waste in intervention research and program planning. Those conducting intervention research through academic institutions need continuous external funding to support themselves and their teams. That means that investigators, interventionists, data analysts, project coordinators, and students are often on to the next project soon after the last data collection period, leaving little time to reflect on findings, carry out discussions with community stakeholders, or use the data collected to gain a deeper understanding of how the intervention worked. Those conducting programs in community health practice have the same funding constraints. Money may be allocated for a specific program but with a limited time frame. Often, when the money and time run out, the program is "done" and the potential to build on lessons learned is minimized as staff are pulled to be on different projects. Investigators should be mindful of the time required to clean and analyze data sets as well as the time required to digest and consider the results. In addition, funders need to be aware of the time required to fully analyze the results of an intervention study and be prepared to continue to fund teams well past the last day of the intervention or final data collection period.

Example of Revising an Intervention: Healthy Teens, Healthy Planet

After a successful pilot that resulted in minor changes to the intervention and evaluation protocol, an RCT was conducted. Twenty schools were randomized to condition, with 10 schools in each condition. Process data showed that the intervention was delivered with fidelity, but there were a few issues with students receiving the intended dose of the classroom component. Absenteeism and a snow day in the middle of the week when the three-session curriculum was to be delivered meant that in several schools, not all students received the full dose of the curricular sessions. Revisions to the intervention protocol will include videotaping the classroom sessions so that they can be viewed outside of the regularly planned delivery time.

The intervention was found to be effective in meeting its goal of reducing students' intake of SSBs by 50% of baseline consumption but moderation analysis found that the effects were stronger in the smaller compared with the larger schools. A mediation analysis found that in smaller schools, the determinants from the social level (descriptive norms, observational learning, and social reinforcements) were significant mediators of the impact of the intervention on SSB consumption. Those effects were not as large in the larger schools; the team wonders whether this diminished effect was due to the larger student body creating less of a singular, strong social network. The intervention team will plan on conducting formative assessment with students and staff at larger schools to better understand how to create more social cohesion and support around healthy beverage choices.

Finally, in the exit interviews with school administration and other community stakeholders, the question of parent involvement was discussed. As the intervention was being implemented, some parents contacted the school to understand why their child's beverage options had changed at school. For the next iteration of the intervention, more attention will be paid to informing parents about the new initiative to decrease student consumption of SSBs through the school's newsletter. The positive results and responses to the program from students and school staff collected through process data will be included in the information as a way to reassure parents that the program has been well received and valued by the school community.

SUMMARY OF THE EVALUATE PHASE

Program evaluation and intervention research requires different skill sets from those required for designing interventions, and the intervention team will need to engage with colleagues who have those skills. Evaluating MLI requires specific skills related to finding robust measurement tools to assess determinants at the individual, social, and physical environment levels. The evaluation requires attention to study design and measurement selection to increase the chance that changes in the behavioral outcome can be attributed to the intervention. For research teams conducting MLIs using group- or cluster-randomized trials, the expertise of biostatisticians will be needed. The importance of the conceptual model, developed earlier in the design process, again becomes evident in the Evaluate Phase because it is used to identify the determinants, behavior, and moderators that will need to be assessed and it also suggests the analytic models to be tested. Teams should do the best they can to learn from each intervention designed and evaluated and be prepared to share their knowledge with others. Ideally, the goal is to create prototypes of effective interventions that are specific to a health behavior change that can be shared with other communities and disseminated or adapted to meet their particular needs. In Chapter 7, I discuss how to use the process described for designing interventions for adapting interventions.

7

Using the Intervention Design Process to Guide the Adaptation of an Evidence-Based Intervention

Although this volume has focused on designing new community-based interventions, many groups will want to adapt existing interventions that have been tested and found to be effective in other communities. Adapting an existing intervention can be more efficient by saving time and costs and can help to disseminate interventions more quickly. Too often, however, interventions that have been found to be effective are abandoned in the communities where they were tested and never disseminated to other settings. This research-to-practice gap is a result of several factors, including (a) interventions not being designed for sustainability and dissemination, (b) the need for frameworks to guide the dissemination of interventions, and (c) lack of guidance on how to adapt an intervention for other communities. The majority of this chapter focuses on the third challenge and uses the phases and steps presented in this volume as a framework to adapt existing interventions. Included as part of the steps are potential sources for identifying evidence-based interventions (EBIs) and using formative assessment to tailor an EBI to a specific community's needs. As an overview of the broader topic of reducing the research-to-practice gap, this chapter begins with a brief discussion of designing interventions for sustainability and dissemination using the RE-AIM and designing for dissemination (D4D) approaches. The chapter also presents implementation science as a source of frameworks to guide the dissemination of effective interventions. It then works through the 12 steps of the intervention design process, explaining how each step might be helpful in making decisions regarding adaptations.

https://doi.org/10.1037/0000292-008
Designing Interventions to Promote Community Health: A Multilevel, Stepwise Approach,
by L. A. Lytle

DESIGNING INTERVENTIONS FOR SUSTAINABILITY AND DISSEMINATION: RE-AIM

It is frequently argued that the reason effective interventions are neither sustained in the communities where they are tested nor disseminated to other communities is because they are not designed with sustainability or dissemination in mind. Rather, intervention research trials often prioritize the goal of establishing that the intervention being tested is responsible for any change that occurs. Trials with a focus on establishing internal validity are called *efficacy trials*, defined as a test of a program under optimal conditions (Flay, 1986). In these types of trials, threats to internal validity are minimized by tight control over the delivery of the intervention and by testing the intervention in a narrowly defined, homogenous population. Once efficacy is determined, the intervention is tested in an effectiveness trial, which is the evaluation of the intervention delivered under real-world conditions (Flay, 1986). Often, however, the move from efficacy to effectiveness is never attempted or is unsuccessful.

Glasgow and others have argued that although this process of moving from efficacy trials to effectiveness trials may be appropriate for medical interventions such as drug trials or new surgical procedures, the process is "fundamentally different from, and at odds with, programs that succeed in population-based effectiveness settings" (Glasgow et al., 2003, p. 1263). Glasgow contended that, from the onset of their creation, interventions designed for population-based settings need to focus on external validity, or the ability of an approach and its related outcomes to generalize to other populations, settings, conditions, and communities.

Glasgow and colleagues have created the RE-AIM evaluation framework as a way to balance both internal and external validity and to better serve the needs of community-based approaches to improve public health. The RE-AIM framework is an acronym for Reach, Efficacy or Effectiveness, Adoption, Implementation, and Maintenance (https://www.re-aim.org) and is applied to both efficacy and effectiveness studies. *Reach* refers to the representativeness of participants and the degree to which individuals approached to participate in the intervention actually participate. *Efficacy or Effectiveness* refers to the impact of the intervention on desired outcomes. *Adoption* operates at a systems level and refers to the proportion and representativeness of organizations, settings, or communities that will engage in or take on the intervention. *Implementation* refers to the degree to which the intervention is delivered as designed, including the fidelity, quality, and consistency of intervention delivery. *Maintenance* refers to the sustainability of individual-level behavior change over time, as well as the institutionalization of the intervention in organizational practice. Paying attention to these five factors during both the early development of an intervention and as it is applied to and evaluated in a broader community increases the chances that the intervention will be able to bridge the research-to-practice gap. In short, community-based interventions need to be designed for dissemination (Brownson et al., 2013).

DESIGNING FOR DISSEMINATION (D4D)

Brownson and colleagues (2013) conducted a survey of scientists involved in dissemination and implementation research with a goal of identifying gaps and areas of improvement. On the basis of their findings and related issues, the authors recommend the following:

1. **Initiating system-level changes,** including how research is funded and incentives for conducting dissemination research, the development of new measurement tools and reporting standards, and improving infrastructure to enhance dissemination possibilities

2. **Initiating process-level changes,** including involving stakeholders as early as possible in dissemination efforts, using audience research as a way to engage key stakeholders, and identifying a framework or theories for dissemination efforts and the appropriate means for delivering messages related to dissemination efforts

3. **Creating products** to identify the appropriate message to communicate, including elements to be documented by interventionists such as effectiveness, cost of implementation and the cost-effectiveness of the disseminated intervention, and the need to develop summaries of the research findings for nonacademic use

The intervention design process described in this volume is congruent with the RE-AIM framework and the imperative to design interventions with an eye toward both internal and external validity, as well as sustainability, and dissemination. Glasgow emphasized the importance of considering the context in which an intervention is delivered and the setting, stakeholders, and individuals the intervention is designed to reach. By using a multilevel approach, attention is paid to changing not only the behaviors of individuals but also the social and physical environments that influence individual choice. Working on intervention approaches to have an impact on the context in which behavior occurs is at the core of multilevel intervention design, necessitating working with community organizations and agencies from the onset of the design process.

Likewise, Glasgow (Glasgow et al., 2003) recommended using participatory research methods to tailor interventions, including "developing one's intervention ideas collaboratively with members of the intended audience (individuals, intervention agents, and organizational decision makers)" (p. 1264). Using a community-engaged approach at each phase of the intervention design process works to increase the chances that the intervention will be efficacious in the short term, will be sustained in the community, and that the lessons learned from one community can be shared and facilitate dissemination of the intervention more broadly (National Cancer Institute, n.d.).

FRAMEWORKS TO GUIDE THE DISSEMINATION OF INTERVENTIONS: IMPLEMENTATION SCIENCE

The field of implementation science has grown out of the recognition that highly effective programs are not disseminated widely, greatly reducing the impact that the intervention can have on public health. Implementation science attempts to bridge the gap between research and practice by developing frameworks to help promote the adoption and integration of EBIs into routine health care and public health settings (Brownson et al., 2017).

Implementation science researchers seek to understand the factors that facilitate or impede the dissemination of effective interventions. As examples, implementation scientists may consider and test alternative strategies to accelerate the adoption of an intervention in a new setting or different community; examine how intervention costs impact dissemination; or examine how the fidelity of an intervention is impacted by dissemination. While intervention researchers focus on outcomes related to change at the individual or organizational level, implementation scientists focus on outcomes that serve as indicators of successful implementation as proximal indicators of the implementation process, or as key intermediate outcomes (or mediators) of measures of effectiveness. Examples of implementation outcomes include acceptability, adoption, feasibility, fidelity, and sustainability (Proctor et al., 2011).

Implementation science uses a variety of frameworks to provide a structure for describing, guiding, analyzing, and evaluating implementation efforts (Moullin et al., 2020). Among the most commonly used frameworks are exploration, preparation, implementation, and sustainment (EPIS; Moullin et al., 2019); the Consolidated Framework for Implementation Research (CFIR; Kirk et al., 2016); Practical, Robust Implementation and Sustainability Model (PRISM; Feldstein & Glasgow, 2008); and Replicating Effective Programs (REP; Rotheram-Borus et al., 2000). A discussion of these frameworks and how they are used to understand dissemination is beyond the scope of this chapter; a robust science related to implementation has grown with the recognized need to bridge the research-to-practice gap (see https://dissemination-implementation.org).

Many applications of implementation science begin with the assumption that the intervention being disseminated has been found to be effective. The term *evidence-based intervention* is used to describe an intervention that has been found to achieve practically important changes in behavioral or environmental conditions using a rigorous evaluation approach (Highfield et al., 2016). It has also been defined as a "health-focused intervention, practice, program, or guideline with evidence demonstrating the ability of the intervention to change a health-related behavior or outcome" (National Cancer Institute, n.d., p. 43). In both definitions, the importance of evidence of effectiveness is the starting point; without such evidence, there is little reason to attempt to disseminate an intervention. Implementation science has also tested hybrid designs that blend design components allowing the evaluation of the effectiveness of a newly developed intervention with an evaluation of its implementation and dissemination potential (Curran et al., 2012).

ADAPTATION AS A NECESSARY PART OF DISSEMINATION

The dissemination of EBIs will likely require some adaptation because communities, populations, and intervention settings differ—sometimes in subtle ways, but other times in more substantial ways (Castro et al., 2004).

Although there is a recognized need to adapt interventions to increase their potential for dissemination (Castro et al., 2004) and models of adaptation have

POTENTIAL AREAS OF MISMATCH BETWEEN EBIs AND THE NEEDS OF SPECIFIC COMMUNITIES

Castro et al. (2004) suggested that there are three primary areas of mismatch between EBIs and the intervention needs of specific communities:

- **Community characteristics:** The community may be different from other populations in which the EBI was evaluated in important ways, including
  - language, ethnicity, socioeconomic status of individuals in the community
  - cultural differences that influence intervention-related beliefs, values, and norms
  - community setting and geographic location (i.e., urban, suburban, rural)
  - mismatch between the determinants targeted for change in the EBI and the determinants that are most relevant to the new community
  - lack of community interest or readiness to participate in the intervention

- **Program delivery options:** The community may not be able to deliver the EBI as planned due to factors such as
  - staffing issues, including not having enough individuals in the community with the required expertise
  - settings issues, including the lack of appropriate and convenient space and places to deliver the intervention
  - feasibility issues related to access, including the lack of availability of child-care or the need for remote delivery options

- **Administrative community factors:** There may be significant differences in administrative community factors, including
  - the lack of infrastructure in the community to support and sustain the intervention
  - limited resources and funding sources for community organizations
  - limited community leadership interest in engaging in the program or intervention

been proposed (Aarons et al., 2012; Center for Substance Abuse Prevention, 2002; Highfield et al., 2016; Lau, 2006; Yu & Seligman, 2002), there is not yet an established approach for adapting EBIs. Ideally, adapting an EBI would start with a deep knowledge of the intervention and the mechanisms (sometimes called "active ingredients") by which it is expected to lead to behavior change. Ideally, a conceptual model and logic model, an intervention protocol manual, and all of the intervention materials used would be available from the teams that developed and evaluated the EBI. These materials would provide important details on the determinants that were chosen as the foci of the change as well as details on intervention strategies, the method of delivery, and the intended dose to be delivered for each strategy. Intervention materials would provide detail on the activities, messages, and examples used in the delivery of the intervention. Ideally, results of the intervention that specify the determinants found to be important mediators of change, the required dose received to effect change, and any significant moderators that were identified would be available. Unfortunately, this type of information is rarely available for those adapting EBIs.

Adaptation may involve an attempt to create a more parsimonious intervention to reduce costs or increase efficiency of its delivery. However, interventions are typically evaluated as a single entity, and often little is known about the elements of the intervention that were particularly potent in driving change. Adaptation risks that those elements most crucial to change (referred to as active ingredients, core elements, or essential elements) may be lost, rendering the adapted intervention ineffective. Active ingredients are the parts of the intervention that have the capacity to bring about change and are defining characteristics of the intervention (Colquhoun et al., 2014).

Maintaining the fidelity of the original intervention while creating an adaptation that better fits the needs of a new community is a tricky balance. The literature refers to this tension as the pull between fidelity and external

WHAT MAKES UP THE ACTIVE INGREDIENTS OF AN INTERVENTION?

The National Cancer Institute (NCI; n.d., p. 11) defined the core components of an intervention as follows:

- **The content of the intervention,** including the components used, the strategies, materials, and approaches used to support intervention strategies

- **How the intervention is delivered,** including the setting of the intervention, who provides the intervention, how those delivering the intervention are trained, and the frequency of contact with interventionists

- **The method used,** including behavior change techniques used to change the individual environment and the approaches for influencing the social and physical environments

TYPES OF ADAPTATIONS

The Framework for Reporting Adaptations and Modifications-Enhanced (FRAME) suggests that modifications of EBIs may occur in content, context, training, and evaluation, and in ways that the intervention is implemented or scaled up (Wiltsey Stirman et al., 2019).

- Change in **content** may include tailoring of messages or activities, removing, adding, or substituting intervention activities, changing the order or sequencing of activities, or shortening or lengthening the intervention.

- Changes in **context** may include modifications to the format of the intervention, the setting in which the intervention is delivered, the personnel involved in implementing the intervention and the population or community targeted by the intervention.

- **Training** may need to be adapted to meet the needs of the staff or community stakeholders who will be delivering the intervention in the new community.

- Change in **evaluation** may include adaptation to enhance the appropriateness of evaluation methods, the feasibility of data collection, the data to collect, and ways to present data to enhance its relevance and utility to the community.

- Modifications related to **implementing** the intervention include changes that result as the EBI is scaled up for broader dissemination, including changes that occur if the EBI becomes commercialized for distribution.

validity (Glasgow et al., 2003). Although intervention trials evaluating the effectiveness of an intervention focus on issues of internal validity (Was the study designed to be able to show a causal relationship between the intervention and the outcome of interest?), adaptation and dissemination of EBIs are a test of the external validity of the intervention (Can the results of the intervention be replicated in other communities?). Implementation science recognizes that adaptation of an EBI may be needed to meet community needs, yet it provides scant direction on how that adaptation should occur. Kilbourne et al. (2007) noted that too often, adapted interventions experience a "voltage drop" in effectiveness and attribute this loss of effectiveness to a loss of fidelity to the original intervention and to the lack of guidance on how to adapt EBI.

CONSIDERATIONS AND GENERAL APPROACHES FOR ADAPTATION

The resource *Implementation Science at a Glance* (NCI, n.d.) provides general guidance for those wishing to adapt an EBI. The authors suggest a "stoplight" approach for considering the appropriateness of adapting an EBI while retaining the active ingredients that drive its effectiveness. Minor changes made to increase the reach, receptivity, and community participation in the program are considered "green-light changes" that can usually be made without the risk of diluting the important active ingredients of the EBI. Examples of green-light changes include changing examples, language, or pictures to make the intervention material more relevant to the new community. "Yellow-light changes" are those that need to be approached with caution because they have the potential to change active ingredients. Examples of yellow-light changes include changing the intervention's delivery mode or format, adding new intervention activities or eliminating existing intervention activities, expanding the primary audience, or changing the sequence of intervention activities. "Red-light changes" should be avoided when possible because of the likelihood of negatively affecting the active ingredients of the original EBI. Red-light changes include changing the health behavior theory or the behavior targeted and tested in the original EBI, eliminating intervention components, reducing the dose of the intervention, and reducing the length of the intervention. If substantial changes to the EBI are made, the effectiveness of the adapted intervention needs to be confirmed through rigorous evaluation.

There are several sources that describe a systematic approach to adaptation. *Implementation Science at a Glance* (NCI, n.d.) suggests that adaptation occurs through a process that includes the following:

1. assessing fit and considering adaptation
2. assessing the acceptability and importance of adaptation
3. making final decisions
4. making adaptations
5. pretesting and piloting test

These steps are part of a process that occurs with the new community to have the intervention better fit the population or local conditions. The more adaptations that are made, the more that pretesting, pilot testing, and additional evaluation are necessary.

Likewise, the Centers for Disease Control and Prevention (CDC; 2006) developed Replicating Effective Programs (REP) as a way to disseminate effective programs, which includes some guidance on adapting EBIs (see also Rotheram-Borus et al., 2000). REP consists of four phases:

1. precondition (e.g., identifying need, target population, and suitable intervention)
2. pre-implementation (e.g., intervention packaging and community input)
3. implementation (e.g., package dissemination, training, technical assistance, and evaluation)
4. maintenance and evolution (e.g., preparing the intervention for sustainability)

The precondition phase includes identifying the need for an intervention in a community and existing EBIs that may fill the need. This phase also includes consideration of the barriers to implementing the EBI in the new community through formative work and ends with a first draft of a revised intervention protocol. The pre-implementation phase includes engaging with community stakeholders to work through issues related to implementation, including training and delivery of the intervention and the creation of a revised intervention protocol or technical manual. A pilot test of the revised EBI is included in this phase, followed by preparation for the implementation phase with the creation of the final REP package, which includes (a) the intervention protocol, (b) all of the intervention materials, and (c) information on staffing needs and electronic files of the intervention and supporting materials. The implementation phase is marked by dissemination of the revised intervention and continues with intervention training, technical assistance, and evaluation. The evaluation includes process evaluation related to how the intervention was delivered and, importantly, an evaluation of fidelity to assess whether the core elements or active ingredients of the EBI were maintained in the adaptation. An outcome evaluation to assess the impact of the adapted intervention on health outcomes and a cost–benefit analysis are also recommended. The last phase of REP is maintenance and evolution, which comprises working with community stakeholders on sustainability, continuing to refine the intervention, and recustomizing the intervention to meet community needs as appropriate (Kilbourne et al., 2007).

The REP process recognizes the need for identifying and maintaining the core elements of the EBI (Kilbourne et al., 2007). The importance of having access to a conceptual model detailing the determinants being addressed; an intervention protocol that specifies content, delivery, and dose of the intervention; the availability of all intervention materials in digital form; training manuals; and a clear a logic model laying out how the intervention activities are operationalized are considered essential for adaptation of an intervention. Without such detail, successful adaptation is threatened. As useful as the REP is, it provides no guidance on how the team adapting the EBI chooses the specific aspects of the intervention to be modified (e.g., specific intervention components, strategies, and related activities and materials) and how those changes are made. Although agencies and scientists interested in disseminating effective programs emphasize the need for a systematic approach for adapting interventions and evaluating adapted interventions, scant attention is paid to how a team chooses the elements of the intervention to be modified or the actual process involved in making changes to the intervention.

APPLYING THE INTERVENTION DESIGN PROCESS TO ADAPTING EBIs

Adapting interventions can be the work of researchers or practitioners. Researchers may be interested in adapting promising or evidence-based interventions and testing their effectiveness in different populations, using rigorous evaluation methods. Their intent may be to evaluate the external validity of an intervention approach. For practitioners, the process of identifying, adapting, and evaluating EBIs may be the primary way that community programs or interventions occur. In an attempt to help with this important step of adaptation for dissemination, the next section describes how researchers and practitioners would use the intervention design process described in this volume to adapt an intervention.

Adapting the Steps From the Plan Phase

Step 1: Identify a Behavior-Based Community Health Problem

The first step, "Identify a behavior-based community health problem," is the starting point for both developing a new intervention and adapting an existing one. Any intervention or program introduced to a community must be in response to some need acknowledged by the community. A community need may be identified when community stakeholders search out health agencies for assistance in solving a recognized community-wide problem. Alternatively, surveillance or other health data may document a community's increased risk for a behaviorally based health threat.

As behaviorally based health risks are identified and the community, health professionals, funders, and other stakeholders prioritize the need for a program to help remediate the risk, EBIs are sought out as possible program options. EBIs may be identified through several sources, including a health agency, funder, supervisor, or recommendations from a colleague. EBIs may be discovered through a conference or continuing education. Often professional groups or societies will create guidelines for specific health threats, and those guidelines include recommended EBIs. As an example, the American Diabetes Association identifies the National Diabetes Prevention Program (CDC, 2021), a CDC-recognized EBI lifestyle intervention program for people with prediabetes, as a program resource for community health workers.

There are also websites that contain information on EBIs. Table 7.1 provides examples of 10 websites created for the purpose of increasing awareness of evidence-based interventions or approaches. The Community Guide to Preventive Medicine (https://thecommunityguide.org) uses systematic reviews and meta-analyses to identify the types of components or intervention strategies that have been found to be effective in leading to behavioral or environmental change. Likewise, the U.S. Preventive Service Task Force (USPSTF; n.d.) is made up of a 16-member volunteer panel of experts in the fields of preventive medicine and primary care that make evidence-based recommendations based on a rigorous review of existing peer-reviewed evidence. Recommendations are published in peer-reviewed journals and provide guidance for practitioners on best practices. Links to those recommendations are provided on the USPSTF website. The Healthy People 2020, Tools and Resources site (Office of Disease Prevention and Health Promotion, 2021) includes an evidence-based database to help practitioners and community stakeholders find interventions and resources to help improve the health of communities. Users can narrow

TABLE 7.1. Examples of Sources for Evidence-Based Intervention Approaches

Source	Provider of information	Type of information
The Community Guide (https://www.thecommunity guide.org/findings)	Community Preventive Services Task Force, CDC	Searchable database that offers a rating of the evidence for various intervention approaches (strong, sufficient, insufficient evidence) and provides links to recommended practices and related rationale
U.S. Preventive Service Task Force (https://uspreventiveservices taskforce.org/uspstf/topic_search_results?topic_status=P)	16-member volunteer panel of experts appointed by the USDHHS	Published recommendations on best practices for intervention approaches based on systematic reviews
Healthy People 2020, Tools and Resources (https://www.healthypeople.gov/2020/tools-resources/Evidence-Based-Resources)	USDHHS	Provides a portal to intervention recommendations made by the CDC's Community Preventive Services Task Force
Canadian Best Practices Portal (https://cbpp-pcpe.phac-aspc.gc.ca/interventions/search-interventions/#)	Public Health Agency of Canada	Classifies interventions as: Best practices, Promising practices, and Aboriginal "Ways Tried and True"; provides an overview of the intervention, contact information for the program developer, link to the intervention site with access to materials, training, and technical assistance
National Association of County and City Health Offices Model Practices (http://www.naccho.org)	Organization serving local health departments	Public health tools, including promising programs, shared by public health practitioners
Pew McArthur First Initiative database (https://www.pewtrusts.org/en/research-and-analysis/data-visualizations/2015/results-first-clearinghouse-database)	Data pulled from nine national clearinghouses	Program's descriptions, outcomes, setting and target population, quality of the intervention rated based on rigor of the evidence
Blueprints for Healthy Youth Development website (http://blueprintsprograms.org)	Institute of Behavioral Sciences at University of Colorado–Boulder	Certify interventions using three categories of evidence; provides a fact sheet with contact information of program developer, description of the program, outcomes, brief evaluation methodology, contact information for program developer, link to materials, training, and technical support availability

(continues)

TABLE 7.1. Examples of Sources for Evidence-Based Intervention Approaches (*Continued*)

Source	Provider of information	Type of information
Substance Abuse and Mental Health Services Administration (http://samhsa.gov)	USDHHS	Listing of model programs related to the prevention of addictive behaviors, guides, evidence reviews, and toolkits for dissemination
HIV Effective Interventions: HIV Prevention That Works (https://www.cdc.gov/hiv/research/interventionresearch/compendium/index.html)	CDC	Descriptions of programs found to be effective for preventing HIV and links to materials and core elements of each program
Evidence-Based Cancer Control Programs (http://ebccp.cancercontrol.cancer.gov)	National Cancer Institute	Listing and rating of evidence-based programs with guaranteed access to materials including contact information for program developer, direct links to intervention materials and training and technical support

Note. CDC = Centers for Disease Control and Prevention; USDHHS = U.S. Department of Health and Human Services.

their search for an intervention by designating a topic area, strength of evidence, population group, race/ethnicity, age, and other criteria. The resource offered is an overview of effective strategies compiled by the CDC's Community Preventive Services Task Force (n.d.).

Similarly, the Public Health Agency of Canada hosts the Canadian Best Practices Portal (n.d.), which classifies existing interventions as Best Practices, Promising Practices, and Aboriginal "Ways Tried and True." Those interventions classified as Best Practices have shown high impact, high adaptability, and high quality of evidence in several trials. This site provides an overview of the EBI and a link to the intervention site where intervention materials and, in some cases, links to technical assistance and training are provided. The National Association of County and City Health Offices (n.d.) Model Practices Program is an award program that recognizes and lists model practice-based programs and toolkits around the country, as well as showcasing promising programs.

The Pew McArthur First Initiative is an online resource that brings together information on the effectiveness of social policy programs, including health interventions related to child and family well-being, mental health, public health, sexual behavior and teen pregnancy, and substance use (Pew Charitable Trusts, 2021). The database pulls information from nine national clearinghouses and includes information on each program's descriptions, outcomes, setting, and target population. They also rate the quality of the intervention based on the rigor of the study.

The Blueprints for Healthy Youth Development (n.d.) website, maintained by the Institute of Behavioral Science at the University of Colorado–Boulder, is a source of EBIs specific to youth development programs. The Blueprints for Healthy Youth Development certifies interventions using three categories: Promising interventions that meet the minimum standard of effectiveness, Model interventions that meet a higher standard and provide greater confidence in the program's ability to change behavior and targeted outcomes, and Model Plus interventions that meet an additional standard of independent replication. In addition to this rating scheme, they provide contact information for the intervention developer, a description of the intervention, outcomes and evaluation methodology, and a link to training and technical support available for replicating the intervention.

The Substance Abuse and Mental Health Services Administration (n.d.) of the U.S. Department of Health and Human Services provides an Evidence-based Practices Resource Center that includes model programs that have been rigorously reviewed and determined to be effective for the prevention of addictive behaviors as well as treatment programs for mental health and substance abuse. The website provides guides, evidence reviews, fact sheets, toolkits, and links to EBI. In another example of a topic-specific intervention site, the CDC hosts a website detailing HIV prevention interventions (CDC, n.d.-c). The website includes descriptions of interventions to treat and prevent HIV as well as links to materials and lists of core elements.

Finally, the U.S. National Cancer Institute (n.d.) maintains the Evidence-Based Cancer Control Programs (EBCCP). The EBCCP includes descriptions of programs published within the past 10 years with guaranteed access to materials. Programs are rated for research integrity, intervention impact, and dissemination capability. In addition, RE-AIM scores are presented for each EBI. Each featured program includes links to or ways to order the intervention materials and contact information for the intervention developer.

These types of websites are an excellent place to begin looking for an appropriate EBI to meet the community's need. While some websites provide details on the intervention, other websites provide only general information (Highfield et al., 2016). Of the websites highlighted in Table 7.1, Canadian Best Practices Portal, Blueprints for Healthy Youth Development, HIV Effective Interventions, and the EBCCP identify core elements of the intervention and provide direct links to the intervention developer, intervention materials, and training and technical support for implementing the intervention. Other websites provide an overview of the types of approaches that have shown some degree of effectiveness, sometimes relying on only one or two rigorous studies and other times based on systematic reviews of the literature. The information available on the website may highlight intervention components that seem to be important for a specific behavioral area but often lack details on intervention implementation. Without details on the behavioral determinants targeted, components included, intervention strategies employed, recommended dose or delivery methods, and active ingredients, adaptation of the EBI delivered with any degree of fidelity to the original EBI is impossible to achieve. However, this general information may provide a first step in examining the types of interventions that have been found to be effective in influencing the health risk of interest and provide the planning group with direction in searching for interventions to adapt.

Before choosing an EBI to use or adapt, the intervention team will need to assess the fit of the EBI with the community's needs and resources. Highfield et al. (2016) suggested three criteria for examining fit:

1. The EBI addresses the same or a similar health problem and the related behaviors and determinants of the behavior used in the EBI match those of the new community.

2. Organizational capacity and resources are available to implement the EBI or a slightly modified version of the EBI.

3. Characteristics of the population evaluated in the EBI are similar to the population for the adapted intervention or the EBI can be modified to accommodate differences in the new population.

Estimating the fit of the health problem and related behaviors should be relatively easy because it is the recognition of a behavior-based health problem that instigates the search for an effective intervention. Likewise, considering fit for the organizational capacity, resources, and the population may be relatively easy by looking at published articles describing the intervention and the sample involved in its evaluation. For example, an EBI using a sophisticated urban media campaign would not likely be considered for a more rural population. Likewise, an EBI requiring many components working across many systems (e.g., a worksite intervention targeting corporate policy, change to the physical environment of the worksite, and on-site health promotion programs) might not be appropriate for a less resourced community.

Community stakeholders need to be involved in the process of identifying appropriate EBIs. In particular, it is important to obtain feedback on how any candidate EBI matches and enhances community capacity. In addition, consideration of the appropriateness of intervention components, delivery methods and possible evaluation strategies is needed. If formative assessment with community stakeholders reveals that the EBI is not appropriate for this population, the EBI should not be used. It is important to keep in mind that sometimes EBIs are copyrighted and, therefore, cannot be modified without the permission of the entity holding the copyright. Teams are advised to check on the copyright status of an intervention before choosing it for adaptation.

Step 2: Choose the Relevant Behavioral Determinants
The second step of the intervention design process involves identifying the determinants targeted in the EBI and matching those with the determinants driving the behavior in the new community. Ideally, an intervention protocol, a conceptual model, and a logic model are available from the original researchers

that provide clarity on the mechanism for change, particularly the behavioral determinants that were targeted. Some websites described in Table 7.1 may provide direct links to those materials. Speaking directly with the original investigators about how the intervention was designed will have many benefits for those adapting it, but often making that direct connection is difficult. For interventions that are funded through the National Institutes of Health (NIH), investigators are required to register their trials on an NIH website, clinicaltrials.gov; this site provides additional detail about the intervention trial and may provide useful information on the mechanisms of the intervention.

If there is no source that clearly identifies the determinants that were targeted in the candidate EBI, the team will need to look to the published literature or professional reports describing the intervention and its outcomes. Outcome papers rarely describe the intervention in sufficient detail to identify the specific determinants targeted. Published papers on secondary outcomes of the trial, an intervention design paper, or a paper on the conceptual model may provide information on the targeted determinants. A published paper describing the mediators of change will be most helpful in seeing how the intervention was intended to affect determinants. A published evaluation report designed for community stakeholders may provide insights into the determinants targeted. If sufficient detail is not available, the team will need to make their best judgments regarding the focus of the intervention by examining the intervention activities, messages, and materials and attempting to discern what factors were being targeted. It may be helpful to consider which environments (individual, social, or physical) were targeted in the EBI and then think of the theoretical constructs that represent those environments (see Chapter 2).

Once a reasonable list of the determinants used in the original EBI is generated, the next adaptation activity is to conduct formative evaluation to better understand how closely the set of determinants targeted in the EBI matches the behavioral determinants for the new community. The formative work can take several shapes. It can focus on surveillance or epidemiologic data specific to the new community—for example, county-level data showing the specific risk factors for prediabetes in a rural community. It can draw on theories that highlight how a specific population experiences health risks—for example, how behavioral health risks of pregnant teens may differ from behavioral health risks of adult women. It can involve collecting qualitative data, asking the target audience and other stakeholders to express their opinions and views on the factors that influence the behavior of interest.

As an example, imagine that formative assessment is being conducted to see if an EBI found to increase children's physical activity levels in neighborhoods in an urban area can be adapted for neighborhoods in suburban areas. The EBI includes two intervention components: (a) increasing neighborhood options for youth to be active (influencing the physical environment) and (b) a family component to encourage children's physical activity (influencing the social environment). A good match between the determinants targeted for

QUESTIONS TO BE ANSWERED DURING FORMATIVE EVALUATION ABOUT THE FIT OF DETERMINANTS

- Are the behavioral determinants targeted in the EBI also relevant to the new community?

- Are there determinants in the EBI that do not apply to the new community or determinants related to the behavior in the new community that are missing from the EBI?

- Are there determinants from the EBI that are relevant to the new population but are expressed differently in the new community?

both urban and suburban areas will increase the team's confidence that the EBI might be a good choice for adaptation. Targeting the same determinants suggests that the intervention objectives, components, and strategies used in the EBI may also apply for the new community, requiring only minor changes (green-light changes) to the EBI. However, the formative assessment may find that some determinants included in the EBI are not relevant to the suburban neighborhoods—for example, the need to change traffic patterns in urban areas to create safe places to play. It may be possible to eliminate some intervention activities targeting irrelevant determinants from an EBI without reducing the effectiveness of the intervention. If an entire component is eliminated, however, it is likely that active ingredients of the EBI will be lost. If many determinants from the EBI are not relevant to the new community, other EBIs should be consider for a better fit.

Alternatively, the formative assessment may show that there are determinants that influence the activity behavior of children in suburban environments that were not included in the urban environment studied in the EBI. For example, the need for transportation to activities may emerge as an important determinant of children's physical activity in the suburban community. The adapted intervention will need to create new intervention objectives, strategies, and approaches for addressing this important determinant. If determinants that are important to the new community are missing from the EBI, the team may look to other interventions that have successfully targeted the missing determinant or may design their own strategies to target the determinant. However, these would be considered yellow-light changes, and their potential impact on the effectiveness would need to be carefully considered. Adding activities or components to an EBI may stretch resources too thin and may weaken the active ingredients of the EBI.

The formative assessment may also reveal a match in determinants, but the determinants are experienced differently in the new community. As an example, the EBI and the new community may both identify parents' perceptions of barriers as a determinant to be addressed in the family component of the intervention, but the types of barriers may differ between groups. The EBI may have identified safety concerns as important perceived barriers related to children's activity levels, while the formative assessment suggests that families in the suburban community perceive a different barrier, a perception that the types or amounts of facilities available in the neighborhood are inadequate. Although "perceived barriers" is the same determinant, the types of barriers differ between groups, and the intervention strategies and approaches, will need to be adapted. If the adaptation needed involves only minimal changes to the intervention materials, then such changes would suggest green-light changes that are not likely to compromise the voltage of the EBI; more substantial changes need to be approached with careful consideration.

Step 3: Create a Conceptual Model

Based on the formative work, the conceptual model may include a mix of all or most of the determinants targeted in the EBI as well as a few additional determinants found to be unique to the behavior of the new community. Grouping determinants by the three environmental levels (individual, social, and physical environments), the team will create a conceptual model that illustrates how the intervention is expected to impact behavior and health outcomes. It is useful to indicate the determinants that were included in the EBI that will and will not continue to be a focus of the intervention and to identify the additional determinants identified through formative work to be targeted in the adapted intervention. This delineation will add transparency regarding how the EBI was adapted and will be helpful in other dissemination efforts of the EBI. A list of potential moderating factors or covariates should also be included in the conceptual model.

Step 4: Review the Conceptual Model With the Evaluation Team and Community Stakeholders

The evaluation goals for intervention teams adapting an EBI may differ from those evaluating newly created interventions; a fully randomized controlled trial (RCT) may not be necessary because the effectiveness of the intervention was already demonstrated. Regardless of the goals, though, some type of evaluation of the adapted EBI will likely occur; the organization sponsoring the intervention work, the funders, and community stakeholders will want to know whether and how the adapted intervention affected their community. To that end, the intervention team should provide the evaluation team published articles and other relevant material they have collected related to the EBI and produce a conceptual model of the adapted intervention to share with the evaluation team and community stakeholders.

Using those materials, the evaluation team should be able to identify the measurement tools and the evaluation protocol originally used to test the EBI.

Often, the evaluation team will need to contact the investigators involved in evaluating the original EBI to get copies of the measurement tools and evaluation protocol or look for other sources of measurement tools as described in the Evaluate Phase (Chapter 6, this volume). In addition, the intervention team will need to highlight the new determinants identified through formative assessment and ask the evaluation team to identify measurement tools to assess change in those determinants. Just as elements of the intervention will need to be adapted to fit the needs of the community, evaluation tools used to test the original EBI may also need to be adapted to make them more culturally appropriate or to more closely match the experience of the community. Recommendations for adapting evaluation tools are just beginning to become available (Foti et al., 2020). Using a similar evaluation plan for the adapted intervention as was used in the EBI helps build the evidence for that intervention contributing to its external validity.

Adapting the Steps From the Create Phase

Steps 5 and 6: Write the Intervention Objectives and Identify Potential Intervention Components; Design Intervention Strategies

Once the conceptual model is revised, it is time to consider how to adapt the intervention components and strategies used by the EBI to enact change. Step 5, "Write the intervention objectives and identify potential intervention components," involves considering the components targeted by the EBI. The screening process for identifying potential EBIs will likely eliminate interventions that used components inappropriate for the new population. Adding or eliminating entire components from the original EBI to be used in the adapted intervention is likely a change that would risk the integrity of the EBI and should be avoided (a red-light change). To eliminate a component for an adapted intervention risks losing the active ingredient of the EBI. To add additional components to an EBI may compromise the resources needed to deliver the original components. If an adaptation involves eliminating or adding components to an EBI, a rigorous evaluation of the adapted intervention using an RCT is recommended to confirm the effectiveness of the adapted approach.

Although it may be possible to modify components, a major adaptation would require careful consideration. For example, it may be possible to adapt a school-based intervention with a curriculum component for an after-school intervention with an educational activities component. Or it may be possible to adapt a clinic-based intervention using motivational interviewing delivered by nurses for a community-based intervention that delivers the motivational interviewing using peer educators in a virtual setting, but these adaptations may dilute the effect of the EBI. The level of expertise that a trained teacher brings to the curriculum and structure of a school class session may not translate to the resources available at a community center and the social environment of an afterschool program. Likewise, the clinic-based approach may work because direct contact with a trained nurse in a clinic system invokes the needed gravitas and personal connection needed to motivate the patient to comply. A virtual adaptation may not be as effective if it lacks those two elements.

Step 6 of the design process is "Design intervention strategies." The most typical type of adaptation that occurs in this phase is to examine the appropriateness of the intervention strategies used and to look for language or examples that need to be adapted to be more culturally appropriate to the new audience. This is a good time for more formative evaluation in which input is received from stakeholders on the specifics of the intervention strategies that were used in the EBI.

Adaptation of the intervention strategies should include a review of the language and examples used throughout the intervention in an effort to make them more appropriate for the population of interest. Simple changes in the words used, changing the names in scenarios, the tone of the writing or illustrations that better reflect the new population may help make the EBI more acceptable to a new community. Different examples may be needed to reflect the new setting or population. For example, adapting an EBI that focuses on changing eating habits for a different culture may require using different foods as examples. Adapting an EBI for a worksite intervention to reduce stress originally designed for a small industrial plant will need different examples if it is being adapted for a business office setting. These changes may be subtle, but they are important in helping make the adapted EBI more accessible and more relevant to a new community or population. Changes to intervention strategies should be minimized to the extent possible because adaptation threatens the integrity of the EBI. In addition, new intervention strategies will need to be designed for any additional determinants identified through formative assessment. New intervention strategies should not require an additional intervention component or a major shift in approach from the EBI.

Steps 7 and 8: Create a Logic Model and Share the Logic Model With the Evaluation Team and Community Stakeholders

The next steps, "Create a logic model" and "Share the logic model with the community and the evaluation team," mirror the process that occurs when

---

QUESTIONS TO BE ANSWERED DURING FORMATIVE EVALUATION ABOUT THE FIT OF INTERVENTION STRATEGIES

- Are the strategies appropriate for the community?
- Are the materials and messages used in these strategies appropriate and engaging for the community?
- Is the requisite expertise to deliver the intervention strategies as designed in the EBI available in the community?
- Will new staff need to be hired, or will additional training for staff or stakeholders need to occur?

designing a new intervention. Creating a logic model concretizes and documents the adaptations that were made by the intervention team and engaged stakeholders. Sharing the logic model with the community provides an opportunity for final input on the adapted intervention and helps ensure that it is appropriate and meets an expressed need of the community. In addition, it is useful to show the adaptations that were made to the original EBI and logic model to be transparent about changes made.

Adapting the Steps From the Implement and Evaluate Phases

Steps 9 and 10: Develop Process Evaluation Measures and Finalize the Intervention Protocol, Training, and Manuals

Step 9 of the design process is "Develop process evaluation measures." To the extent possible, use the same process measures that were used in the EBI because doing so will provide a direct comparison with how the intervention was delivered and received between the EBI and the adapted intervention. Process measures are also key to understanding how the adapted intervention morphs as it is being disseminated and how robust the intervention implementation is in an adapted version. Data collected on the reach of the intervention will provide important information on the new community's response to and engagement with the adapted EBI. Process data related to fidelity should assess the degree to which the adapted intervention matches the EBI as well as the degree to which the adapted intervention protocol is implemented with fidelity. Likewise, when finalizing the intervention protocol, training, and manuals (Step 10), use as much as possible from the original EBI, both to stay true to the EBI and to take advantage of the resources saved by using a tested EBI. Be clear about the changes made to the EBI in the intervention protocol so that comparisons between the original EBI and its adaptation can be made.

FRAME recommends that those adapting EBI provide detail on the adaptation process, including the intent or rationale for the adaptation and whether the adaptation was made before testing the EBI in a new community or the need for adaptation was instigated by unanticipated obstacles in the intervention process. In addition, they recommend detailed information on the content that was modified, any changes to the delivery of the intervention, and the extent to which the modification is fidelity-consistent—or how similar in approach is the adapted intervention to the original EBI (Baumann et al., 2017; Wiltsey Stirman et al., 2019).

Steps 11 and 12: Evaluate the Effectiveness of the Intervention and Prepare for the Next Iteration or Dissemination of the Intervention

The evaluation goals for an adapted EBI may differ for a practice group compared with a research group. For a community practice group, the choice of an EBI likely reflects an assumption that the intervention has already proven to be effective, and being able to spend less money on a sophisticated evaluation may be a primary impetus for a community agency to choose an EBI. However, some level of evaluation will still be needed because the community will want to know if the intervention worked in their community and be able to answer the following questions:

- Was this adapted EBI, tested in this community, successful in achieving important behavior change?

- Was this adapted EBI, tested in this community, successful in changing the determinants targeted by the intervention?

- Within the population participating in this intervention and evaluation, were there subgroups for whom the intervention worked particularly well or not as well?

At the very least, the use of a pre–post evaluation, examining both change in behavioral and health outcomes and determinants targeted by the adapted EBI, should be conducted. If a pre–post design is used, be aware of its limitations. Without a control or comparison group, it is difficult to confidently attribute change over time to the effect of the intervention. It may also be possible to use a pragmatic design such as a delayed intervention or a stepped wedge design to make comparisons between groups receiving and not receiving the intervention. With a delayed intervention design, two groups are identified to participate in the intervention, and both groups have baseline data collected. One group receives the intervention first and the second group receives a delayed offering of the intervention; both groups are assessed at the end of the first intervention offering. The delayed group serves as a comparison group for the group receiving the intervention. A stepped wedge design begins with an initial period in which baseline data are collected on all the groups or clusters of individuals participating in the trial. At regular intervals, clusters are randomized into the intervention group until all the clusters are exposed to the intervention and data collected on groups exposed and not exposed to the intervention (Hemming et al., 2015).

Researchers may want to test the effectiveness of an adapted intervention using an RCT. This would be especially important if the EBI was adapted for a population that is significantly different from the population evaluated in the original EBI or if major changes were made in the content or delivery of the intervention. As EBIs are adapted, rigorously evaluated, and found to be effective in a wide variety of settings with different populations, the external validity of the intervention approach is established, and the evidence base expands. The next section describes how one research team adapted and evaluated an EBI.

AN EXAMPLE OF ADAPTING AN EBI FOR PREVENTING DATING ABUSE

Families for Safe Dates (FSD) is a family-based dating abuse prevention program that was found to be effective in reducing dating abuse in the general population (Foshee et al., 1998). The intervention involves six booklets mailed to the home with dating abuse prevention information and activities for parents and their adolescents to do together. An RCT found that the intervention was effective in preventing dating abuse victimization, with those adolescents not participating in the program reporting significantly higher rates of victimization as compared with those adolescents participating in the program (Foshee et al., 2012). FSD is recognized as a EBI and is distributed nationally and globally by the Hazelden Publishing and Educational Services.

The creators of FSD saw a need to adapt the program for a higher risk population: children who have been exposed to domestic violence (Foshee, Dixon, et al., 2015). The rationale for an adapted program was the recognition that adolescents who have been exposed to domestic violence are at increased risk for being victims of violence (O'Donnell et al., 2006) and the belief that the parent-based approach of FSD would need to be modified because of sensitivity related to shared violence between participating parent and child. The adapted program was called Moms and Teens for Safe Dates (MTSD) and was designed to be offered to moms and teens who experienced domestic violence but no longer live with the abuser.

The need for a behavioral program to reduce dating violence for youth exposed to domestic violence was verified through surveillance data; approximately 15 million children each year are exposed to domestic violence (McDonald et al., 2006). The original developers of FSD had developed a conceptual model positing that the determinants of psychological, physical, cyber, and sexual dating abuse victimization and perpetration were factors operating at both the mother and teen levels. Their process for adapting FSD began by reviewing the conceptual model and making adjustments based on what theory and evidence suggested were determinants and other factors unique to those experiencing domestic violence. As examples, there was a belief that mothers who had already experienced domestic violence may be particularly attuned to the issue. Therefore, they may not need more information about the risks of dating violence and likely already believed that dating violence was serious and that their teen was susceptible to it. Therefore, they eliminated those constructs from the revised conceptual model for MTSD. In addition, they added a new construct to the model, gender stereotyping, because of empirical evidence suggesting the traditional gender stereotyping is reinforced by witnessing domestic violence.

Next, they revised the content of the six booklets to reflect the changes in the conceptual model. Activities related to increasing knowledge about the risks of dating violence and to increase mothers' perceptions of the severity of dating violence and their child's susceptibility to violence were deleted from the content. Likewise, new content was added to the booklets to push back against adolescent acceptance of traditional gender stereotypes. To further adapt the program to this high-risk audience, the booklets were edited to acknowledge the challenges that the mothers might have participating in the program with their teen because of their previous experience with domestic violence and to congratulate the mothers on their efforts to leave an abusive partner (Foshee, Dixon, et al., 2015).

The formative assessment, including focus groups and interviews, followed this initial redraft of the booklets and occurred with 28 mothers and their adolescent children recruited from community agencies and judicial districts. Mother–child dyads completed booklets together and then participated in a focus group or interview to provide feedback. The focus group and interview guides were designed to assess program comprehension, relevance to the target population, and motivation for doing the booklet activities. In addition, participants were asked to respond to questions about the organization, content, and approach of the material presented in each booklet (Foshee, Dixon, et al., 2015).

The results of the formative evaluation confirmed that the delivery method for the intervention (booklets mailed home with activities designed to facilitate conversation between mother and child) was appropriate and a welcome resource for this at-risk audience. However, they also found that some of their assumptions about changes to be made for this at-risk group were erroneous. They learned that many mothers did not realize dating abuse could begin so early or that their child was at risk for dating abuse. They also heard mothers express a strong desire for more information about psychological abuse because many saw their abusive physical relationships begin with psychological abuse. With this understanding, the investigators added back information regarding the knowledge and severity of dating abuse and adolescents' susceptibility to abuse into the content and added additional content related to psychological abuse. The conceptual model was adjusted to reflect those changes, and the content of the booklet was revised to incorporate this feedback. The MTSD intervention was subsequently evaluated in an RCT and found to be effective in reducing the risk of psychological, physical, and cyber-dating abuse in those teens who had experienced greater exposure to domestic violence. There were no program effects for teens who had experienced little or moderate exposure to violence (Foshee, Benefield, et al., 2015).

SUMMARY OF THE ADAPTATION PROCESS

A systematic approach for adapting EBIs is greatly needed. This need is closely linked with an imperative for intervention designers to create and be prepared to share an intervention protocol, conceptual model, logic model, materials, and evaluation protocol, including outcome and process evaluation methods and data collection forms. Without a clear understanding of how an intervention was designed to create change and the active ingredients involved in that change, there is little chance that an adaptation will be successful. The process of adapting an intervention requires a commitment to finding the best-fitting EBI for the community's health needs and characteristics. Adaptation also requires a systematic approach to confirm or modify the behavioral determinants for the new community, maximize the fidelity to the original EBI, and be clear and transparent about the modifications made. In addition, there is a great need to provide information related to how and why adaptations to

EBIs occur. Only through this careful process and detailed reporting of adaption will the research-to-practice gap be reduced and the dissemination of effective interventions increase.

CONCLUSION

The first step in disseminating effective interventions to promote community health is designing interventions that are effective in creating behavior change. The four-phase, 12-step intervention process described in this volume works toward the objectives of designing interventions that are effective in promoting community health and creating interventions that are designed for sustainability and dissemination. These multiple objectives are accomplished by engaging communities in all phases of the design process and, through that engagement, keeping the intervention grounded in addressing communities' need, building community capacity, and working in more genuine and respectful partnerships with communities. This level of community engagement is important not only for creating effective interventions but also for increasing the chance that the interventions will be relevant to other communities. In addition, interventions that are multilevel have an increased chance of leading to sustained behavior change and work toward building system-level change that can enhance the health of all communities and populations. By using an intervention design process that is systematic, evidence based, and transparent and that uses evaluation methods that allow us to maximize what can be learned, the number of EBIs will grow. And with that growth comes the potential for healthier communities.

REFERENCES

Aarons, G. A., Green, A. E., Palinkas, L. A., Self-Brown, S., Whitaker, D. J., Lutzker, J. R., Silovsky, J. F., Hecht, D. B., & Chaffin, M. J. (2012). Dynamic adaptation process to implement an evidence-based child maltreatment intervention. *Implementation Science*, *7*(1), 32. https://doi.org/10.1186/1748-5908-7-32

Ahmed, S. M., & Palermo, A. G. (2010). Community engagement in research: Frameworks for education and peer review. *American Journal of Public Health*, *100*(8), 1380–1387. https://doi.org/10.2105/AJPH.2009.178137

Ajzen, I. (1991). The theory of planned behavior. *Organizational Behavior and Human Decision Processes*, *50*(2), 179–211. https://doi.org/10.1016/0749-5978(91)90020-T

Aveyard, P., Cheng, K. K., Almond, J., Sherratt, E., Lancashire, R., Lawrence, T., Griffin, C., & Evans, O. (1999). Cluster randomised controlled trial of expert system based on the transtheoretical ("stages of change") model for smoking prevention and cessation in schools. *British Medical Journal*, *319*(7215), 948–953. https://doi.org/10.1136/bmj.319.7215.948

Ball, S. (2008). *The education debate*. The Policy Press.

Bandura, A. (1986). *Social foundations of thought and action: A social cognitive theory*. Prentice Hall.

Baranowski, T., & Stables, G. (2000). Process evaluations of the 5-a-day projects. *Health Education & Behavior*, *27*(2), 157–166. https://doi.org/10.1177/109019810002700202

BaRoss, C. (2017, January 24). *Designing for health: The power of the charrette*. Contract Design Network. https://contractdesign.com/practice/healthcare/Designing-for-Health-The-Power-of-the-Charrette/

Basch, C. E., Sliepcevich, E. M., Gold, R. S., Duncan, D. F., & Kolbe, L. J. (1985). Avoiding Type III errors in health education program planning evaluations:

A case study. *Health Education Quarterly, 12*(3), 315–331. https://doi.org/10.1177/109019818501200311

Bauer, K. W., Neumark-Sztainer, D., Fulkerson, J. A., Hannan, P. J., & Story, M. (2011). Familial correlates of adolescent girls' physical activity, television use, dietary intake, weight, and body composition. *The International Journal of Behavioral Nutrition and Physical Activity, 8*(1), 25. https://doi.org/10.1186/1479-5868-8-25

Baumann, A., Cabassa, I. J., & Sireman, S. W. (2017). Adaptation in dissemination and implementation science. In R. C. Brownson, F. A. Colditz, & E. K. Proctor (Eds.), *Dissemination and implementation research in health: Translating science to practice* (Vol. 2, pp. 286–300). Oxford University Press.

Becker, M. H. (1974). The health belief model and personal health behavior. *Health Education Monographs, 2*(4), 409–419. https://doi.org/10.1177/109019817400200407

Begg, C., Cho, M., Eastwood, S., Horton, R., Moher, D., Olkin, I., Pitkin, R., Rennie, D., Schulz, K. F., Simel, D., & Stroup, D. F. (1996). Improving the quality of reporting of randomized controlled trials: The CONSORT statement. *Journal of the American Medical Association, 276*(8), 637–639. https://doi.org/10.1001/jama.1996.03540080059030

Béland, D., & Howlett, M. (2016). The role and impact of the Multiple-Streams Approach in comparative policy analysis. *Journal of Comparative Policy Analysis, 18*(3), 221–227. https://doi.org/10.1080/13876988.2016.1174410

Birnbaum, A. S., Lytle, L. A., Story, M., Perry, C. L., & Murray, D. M. (2002). Are differences in exposure to a multicomponent school-based intervention associated with varying dietary outcomes in adolescents? *Health Education & Behavior, 29*(4), 427–443. https://doi.org/10.1177/109019810202900404

Blitstein, J. L., Murray, D. M., Lytle, L. A., Birnbaum, A. S., & Perry, C. L. (2005). Predictors of violent behavior in an early adolescent cohort: Similarities and differences across genders. *Health Education & Behavior, 32*(2), 175–194. https://doi.org/10.1177/1090198104269516

Blueprints for Healthy Youth Development. (n.d.). *Providing a registry of experimentally proven programs.* https://www.blueprintsprograms.org/

Blum, J. E. W., Davee, A. M., Beaudoin, C. M., Jenkins, P. L., Kaley, L. A., & Wigand, D. A. (2008). Reduced availability of sugar-sweetened beverages and diet soda has a limited impact on beverage consumption patterns in Maine high school youth. *Journal of Nutrition Education and Behavior, 40*(6), 341–347. https://doi.org/10.1016/j.jneb.2007.12.004

Bracht, N. (Ed.). (1990). *Health promotion at the community level.* Sage Publications.

Bronfenbrenner, U. (1992). Ecological systems theory. In R. Vasta (Ed.), *Six theories of child development: Revised formulations and current issues* (pp. 187–249). Jessica Kingsley Publishers.

Brownson, R. C., Colditz, G. A., & Proctor, E. K. (Eds.). (2017). *Dissemination and implementation research in health: Translating science to practice* (2nd ed.). Oxford University Press. https://doi.org/10.1093/oso/9780190683214.001.0001

Brownson, R. C., Jacobs, J. A., Tabak, R. G., Hoehner, C. M., & Stamatakis, K. A. (2013). Designing for dissemination among public health researchers: Findings from a national survey in the United States. *American Journal of Public Health, 103*(9), 1693–1699. https://doi.org/10.2105/AJPH.2012.301165

Brownson, R. C., Tabak, R. G., Stamatis, K. A., & Glanz, K. (2015). Implementation, dissemination, and diffusion of public health interventions. In K. Glanz,

B. Rimer, & K. Viswanath (Eds.), *Health behavior: Theory, research and practice* (5th ed., pp. 301–326). Jossey-Bass.

Byrne, R. M. J. (2005). *The rational imagination: How people create counterfactual alternatives to reality*. MIT Press. https://doi.org/10.7551/mitpress/5756.001.0001

Campbell, M. K., Piaggio, G., Elbourne, D. R., Altman, D. G., & the CONSORT Group. (2012). Consort 2010 statement: Extension to cluster randomised trials. *British Medical Journal, 345*, e5661. https://doi.org/10.1136/bmj.e5661

Canadian Best Practices Portal. (n.d.). https://cbpp-pcpe.phac-aspc.gc.ca/interventions/search-interventions/#

Carbon Trust. (2012). *Footprint manager* (Version 4.0) [Computer software]. https://www.carbontrust.com/resources/carbon-footprinting-software

Castro, F. G., Barrera, M., Jr., & Martinez, C. R., Jr. (2004). The cultural adaptation of prevention interventions: Resolving tensions between fidelity and fit. *Prevention Science, 5*(1), 41–45. https://doi.org/10.1023/B:PREV.0000013980.12412.cd

Catalani, C., & Minkler, M. (2010). Photovoice: A review of the literature in health and public health. *Health Education & Behavior, 37*(3), 424–451. https://doi.org/10.1177/1090198109342084

Center for Substance Abuse Prevention. (2002). *Finding the balance: Program fidelity and adaptation in substance abuse prevention: Executive summary of a state-of-the-art review*. U.S. Department of Health and Human Services, Substance Abuse and Mental Health Services Administration. https://www.enap.ca/cerberus/files/nouvelles/documents/CREVAJ/Baker_2002.pdf

Centers for Disease Control and Prevention. (n.d.-a). *Behavioral risk factor surveillance system*. https://www.cdc.gov/brfss/index.html

Centers for Disease Control and Prevention. (n.d.-b). *Community health assessment & health improvement planning*. https://www.cdc.gov/publichealthgateway/cha/index.html

Centers for Disease Control and Prevention. (n.d.-c). *Effective interventions*. https://www.cdc.gov/hiv/effective-interventions/index.html

Centers for Disease Control and Prevention. (n.d.-d). *Surgeon general's reports on smoking and tobacco use*. https://www.cdc.gov/tobacco/data_statistics/sgr/

Centers for Disease Control and Prevention. (n.d.-e). *Youth Risk Behavior Surveillance System (YRBSS)*. https://www.cdc.gov/healthyyouth/data/yrbs/index.htm

Centers for Disease Control and Prevention. (2006). *Replicating effective programs plus*. https://www.cdc.gov/hiv/research/interventionresearch/rep/index.html

Centers for Disease Control and Prevention. (2011). *Introduction to program evaluation for public health programs: A self-study guide*. https://www.cdc.gov/eval/guide/CDCEvalManual.pdf

Centers for Disease Control and Prevention. (2018). *State indicator report on fruits and vegetables, 2018*. https://www.cdc.gov/nutrition/data-statistics/2018-state-indicator-report-fruits-vegetables.html

Centers for Disease Control and Prevention. (2021, August 27). *National Diabetes Prevention Program*. https://www.cdc.gov/diabetes/prevention/index.html

Centers for Disease Control and Prevention, Agency for Toxic Substances and Disease Registry. (1997). *Principles of community engagement*.

Centers for Disease Control and Prevention, Committee on Community Engagement. (1997). *Principles of community engagement*.

Centers for Disease Control and Prevention, Division for Heart Disease and Stroke Prevention. (2003). *Evaluation guide: Developing and using a logic model*. U.S.

Department of Health and Human Services. https://www.cdc.gov/dhdsp/docs/logic_model.pdf

Chan, A. W., Tetzlaff, J. M., Gøtzsche, P. C., Altman, D. G., Mann, H., Berlin, J. A., Dickersin, K., Hróbjartsson, A., Schulz, K. F., Parulekar, W. R., Krleza-Jeric, K., Laupacis, A., & Moher, D. (2013). SPIRIT 2013 explanation and elaboration: Guidance for protocols of clinical trials. *British Medical Journal, 346*, e7586. https://doi.org/10.1136/bmj.e7586

Christakis, N. A., & Fowler, J. H. (2007). The spread of obesity in a large social network over 32 years. *The New England Journal of Medicine, 357*(4), 370–379. https://doi.org/10.1056/NEJMsa066082

Clauser, S. B., Taplin, S. H., Foster, M. K., Fagan, P., & Kaluzny, A. D. (2012). Multi-level intervention research: Lessons learned and pathways forward. *JNCI Monographs, 2012*(44), 127–133. https://doi.org/10.1093/jncimonographs/lgs019

Cleary, P. D., Gross, C. P., Zaslavsky, A. M., & Taplin, S. H. (2012). Multilevel interventions: Study design and analysis issues. *JNCI Monographs, 2012*(44), 49–55. https://doi.org/10.1093/jncimonographs/lgs010

Colquhoun, H., Leeman, J., Michie, S., Lokker, C., Bragge, P., Hempel, S., McKibbon, K. A., Peters, G.-J. Y., Stevens, K. R., Wilson, M. G., & Grimshaw, J. (2014). Towards a common terminology: A simplified framework of interventions to promote and integrate evidence into health practices, systems, and policies. *Implementation Science, 9*, 51. https://doi.org/10.1186/1748-5908-9-51

Community Preventive Services Task Force. (n.d.). *Community Preventive Services Task Force findings*. https://www.thecommunityguide.org/findings

Compton, W. M., Conway, K. P., Stinson, F. S., & Grant, B. F. (2006). Changes in the prevalence of major depression and comorbid substance use disorders in the United States between 1991–1992 and 2001–2002. *The American Journal of Psychiatry, 163*(12), 2141–2147. https://doi.org/10.1176/ajp.2006.163.12.2141

Curran, G. M., Bauer, M., Mittman, B., Pyne, J. M., & Stetler, C. (2012). Effectiveness-implementation hybrid designs: Combining elements of clinical effectiveness and implementation research to enhance public health impact. *Medical Care, 50*(3), 217–226. https://doi.org/10.1097/MLR.0b013e3182408812

de Bruin, M., Black, N., Javornik, N., Viechtbauer, W., Eisma, M. C., Hartman-Boyce, J., Williams, A. J., West, R., Michie, S., & Johnston, M. (2021). Under-reporting of the active content of behavioural interventions: A systematic review and meta-analysis of randomised trials of smoking cessation interventions. *Health Psychology Review, 15*(2), 195–213. https://doi.org/10.1080/17437199.2019.1709098

Donner, A., Taljaard, M., & Klar, N. (2007). The merits of breaking the matches: A cautionary tale. *Statistics in Medicine, 26*(9), 2036–2051. https://doi.org/10.1002/sim.2662

Drummond, R. J., Sheperis, C. J., & Jones, K. D. (2016). *Assessment procedures for counselors and helping professionals* (8th ed.). Pearson.

Dwyer-Lindgren, L., Bertozzi-Villa, A., Stubbs, R. W., Morozoff, C., Mackenbach, J. P., van Lenthe, F. J., Mokdad, A. H., & Murray, C. J. L. (2017). Inequalities in life expectancy among US counties, 1980–2014: Temporal trends and key drivers. *JAMA Internal Medicine, 177*(7), 1003–1011. https://doi.org/10.1001/jamainternmed.2017.0918

Earp, J. A., & Ennett, S. T. (1991). Conceptual models for health education research and practice. *Health Education Research, 6*(2), 163–171. https://doi.org/10.1093/her/6.2.163

Elder, J. P., Lytle, L., Sallis, J. F., Young, D. R., Steckler, A., Simons-Morton, D., Stone, E., Jobe, J. B., Stevens, J., Lohman, T., Webber, L., Pate, R., Saksvig, B. I., & Ribisl, K. (2007). A description of the social-ecological framework used in the trial of activity for adolescent girls (TAAG). *Health Education Research, 22*(2), 155–165. https://doi.org/10.1093/her/cyl059

Elias, R. R., Jutte, D. P., & Moore, A. (2019). Exploring consensus across sectors for measuring the social determinants of health [erratum at https://doi.org/10.1016/j.ssmph.2020.100710]. *SSM—Population Health, 7,* 100395. https://doi.org/10.1016/j.ssmph.2019.100395

Ezendam, N. P. M., Evans, A. E., Stigler, M. H., Brug, J., & Oenema, A. (2010). Cognitive and home environmental predictors of change in sugar-sweetened beverage consumption among adolescents. *British Journal of Nutrition, 103*(5), 768–774. https://doi.org/10.1017/S0007114509992297

Feldstein, A. C., & Glasgow, R. E. (2008). A practical, robust implementation and sustainability model (PRISM) for integrating research findings into practice. *Joint Commission Journal on Quality and Patient Safety, 34*(4), 228–243. https://doi.org/10.1016/S1553-7250(08)34030-6

Fell, J. C., & Voas, R. B. (2006). Mothers Against Drunk Driving (MADD): The first 25 years. *Traffic Injury Prevention, 7*(3), 195–212. https://doi.org/10.1080/15389580600727705

Fishbein, M., & Ajzen, I. (2010). *Predicting and changing behavior: The reasoned action approach.* Psychology Press.

Fisher, E. B., Ballesteros, J., Bhushan, N., Coufal, M. M., Kowitt, S. D., McDonough, A. M., Parada, H., Robinette, J. B., Sokol, R. L., Tang, P. Y., & Urlaub, D. (2015). Key features of peer support in chronic disease prevention and management. *Health Affairs, 34*(9), 1523–1530. https://doi.org/10.1377/hlthaff.2015.0365

Flay, B. R. (1986). Efficacy and effectiveness trials (and other phases of research) in the development of health promotion programs. *Preventive Medicine, 15*(5), 451–474. https://doi.org/10.1016/0091-7435(86)90024-1

Foshee, V. A., Bauman, K. E., Arriaga, X. B., Helms, R. W., Koch, G. G., & Linder, G. F. (1998). An evaluation of Safe Dates, an adolescent dating violence prevention program. *American Journal of Public Health, 88*(1), 45–50. https://doi.org/10.2105/AJPH.88.1.45

Foshee, V. A., Benefield, T., Dixon, K. S., Chang, L. Y., Senkomago, V., Ennett, S. T., Moracco, K. E., & Bowling, M. J. (2015). The effects of moms and teens for safe dates: A dating abuse prevention program for adolescents exposed to domestic violence. *Journal of Youth and Adolescence, 44*(5), 995–1010. https://doi.org/10.1007/s10964-015-0272-6

Foshee, V. A., Dixon, K. S., Ennett, S. T., Moracco, K. E., Bowling, J. M., Chang, L., & Moss, J. L. (2015). The process of adapting universal dating abuse prevention program to adolescents exposed to domestic violence. *Journal of Interpersonal Violence, 30*(12), 2151–2173. https://doi.org/10.1177/0886260514552278

Foshee, V. A., McNaughton Reyes, H. L., Ennett, S. T., Cance, J. D., Bauman, K. E., & Bowling, J. M. (2012). Assessing the effects of Families for Safe Dates, a family-based teen dating abuse prevention program. *The Journal of Adolescent Health, 51*(4), 349–356. https://doi.org/10.1016/j.jadohealth.2011.12.029

Foti, K. E., Perez, C. L., Knapp, E. A., Kharmats, A. Y., Sharfman, A. S., Arteaga, S. S., Moore, L. V., & Bennett, W. L. (2020). Identification of measurement needs to prevent childhood obesity in high-risk populations and environments. *American Journal of Preventive Medicine, 59*(5), 746–754. https://doi.org/10.1016/j.amepre.2020.05.012

Fowler, F. J., Jr. (2014). *Survey research methods* (5th ed.). Sage Publications.

Fulkerson, J. A., Nelson, M. C., Lytle, L., Moe, S., Heitzler, C., & Pasch, K. E. (2008). The validation of a home food inventory. *The International Journal of Behavioral Nutrition and Physical Activity, 5*(1), 55. https://doi.org/10.1186/1479-5868-5-55

Giskes, K., Van Lenthe, F. J., Brug, J., Mackenbach, J. P., & Turrell, G. (2007). Socioeconomic inequalities in food purchasing: The contribution of respondent-perceived and actual (objectively measured) price and availability of foods. *Preventive Medicine, 45*(1), 41–48. https://doi.org/10.1016/j.ypmed.2007.04.007

Glanz, K., & Ammerman, A. (2015). Introduction to community and group models of health behavior change. In K. Glanz, B. Rimer, & K. Viswanath (Eds.), *Health behavior: Theory, research, and practice* (5th ed., pp. 271–277). Jossey-Bass.

Glanz, K., Rimer, B. K., & Viswanath, K. (Eds.). (2015a). *Health behavior: Theory, research, and practice* (5th ed.). Jossey-Bass.

Glanz, K., Rimer, B. K., & Viswanath, K. (Eds.). (2015b). Theory, research, and practice in health behavior. In K. Glanz, B. K. Rimer, & K. Viswanath (Eds.), *Health behavior: Theory, research, and practice* (5th ed., pp. 23–42). Jossey-Bass.

Glasgow, R. E., Lichtenstein, E., & Marcus, A. C. (2003). Why don't we see more translation of health promotion research to practice? Rethinking the efficacy-to-effectiveness transition. *American Journal of Public Health, 93*(8), 1261–1267. https://doi.org/10.2105/AJPH.93.8.1261

Goodman, R. M., Speers, M. A., McLeroy, K., Fawcett, S., Kegler, M., Parker, E., Smith, S. R., Sterling, T. D., & Wallerstein, N. (1998). Identifying and defining the dimensions of community capacity to provide a basis for measurement. *Health Education & Behavior, 25*(3), 258–278. https://doi.org/10.1177/109019819802500303

Goodstadt, M. (2005). *The use of logic models in health promotion practice.* https://institute.welcoa.org/wp/wp-content/uploads/2016/04/Goodstadt-Logic-Models.pdf

Gorin, S. S., Badr, H., Krebs, P., & Prabhu Das, I. (2012). Multilevel interventions and racial/ethnic health disparities. *JNCI Monographs, 2012*(44), 100–111. https://doi.org/10.1093/jncimonographs/lgs015

Gray, H. L., Contento, I. R., Koch, P. A., & di Noia, J. (2016). Mediating mechanisms of theory-based psychosocial determinants on behavioral changes in a middle school obesity risk reduction curriculum intervention, Choice, Control, and Change. *Childhood Obesity, 12*(5), 348–359. https://doi.org/10.1089/chi.2016.0003

Grembowski, D. (2016). *The practice of health program evaluation* (2nd ed.). Sage Publishing.

Hawe, P. (2015). Lessons from complex interventions to improve health. *Annual Review of Public Health, 36*(1), 307–323. https://doi.org/10.1146/annurev-publhealth-031912-114421

Hecht, M. L., & Krieger, J. L. (2006). The principal of cultural grounding in school-based substance abuse prevention: The Drug Resistant Strategies Project. *Journal of Language and Social Psychology, 25*(3), 301–319. https://doi.org/10.1177/0261927X06289476

Hemming, K., Haines, T. P., Chilton, P. J., Girling, A. J., & Lilford, R. J. (2015). The stepped wedge cluster randomised trial: Rationale, design, analysis, and reporting. *British Medical Journal, 350*, h391. https://doi.org/10.1136/bmj.h391

Highfield, L., Hartman, M. A., Mullen, P. D., & Leelooijer, J. N. (2016). Using intervention mapping to adapt evidence-based interventions. In L. K. Bartholomew Eldredge, C. M. Markham, R. A. C. Ruiter, M. E. Fernández, G. Kok, & G. S. Parcel. *Planning health promotion programs: An intervention mapping approach* (4th ed., pp. 597–649). Jossey-Bass.

Hoelscher, D. M., Feldman, H. A., Johnson, C. C., Lytle, L. A., Osganian, S. K., Parcel, G. S., Kelder, S. H., Stone, E. J., & Nader, P. R. (2004). School-based health education programs can be maintained over time: Results from the CATCH Institutionalization study. *Preventive Medicine, 38*(5), 594–606. https://doi.org/10.1016/j.ypmed.2003.11.017

Hoffmann, T. C., Erueti, C., & Glasziou, P. P. (2013). Poor description of non-pharmacological interventions: Analysis of consecutive sample of randomised trials. *British Medical Journal, 347*, f3755. https://doi.org/10.1136/bmj.f3755

Hoffmann, T. C., Glasziou, P. P., Boutron, I., Milne, R., Perera, R., Moher, D., Altman, D. G., Barbour, V., Macdonald, H., Johnston, M., Lamb, S. E., Dixon-Woods, M., McCulloch, P., Wyatt, J. C., Chan, A. W., & Michie, S. (2014). Better reporting of interventions: Template for intervention description and replication (TIDieR) checklist and guide. *British Medical Journal, 348*, g1687. https://doi.org/10.1136/bmj.g1687

Holt-Lunstad, J., & Uchino, B. N. (2015). Social support and health. In K. Glanz, B. K. Rimer, & K. Viswanath (Eds.), *Health behavior: Theory, research, and practice* (5th ed., pp. 183–201). Jossey-Bass.

Hopfer, S., & Clippard, J. R. (2011). College women's HPV vaccine decision narratives. *Qualitative Health Research, 21*(2), 262–277. https://doi.org/10.1177/1049732310383868

Humphrey, S. E., & LeBreton, J. M. (Eds.). (2019). *The handbook of multilevel theory, measurement, and analysis*. American Psychological Association. https://doi.org/10.1037/0000115-000

Janega, J. B., Murray, D. M., Varnell, S. P., Blitstein, J. L., Birnbaum, A. S., & Lytle, L. A. (2004a). Assessing intervention effects in a school-based nutrition intervention trial: Which analytic model is most powerful? *Health Education & Behavior, 31*(6), 756–774. https://doi.org/10.1177/1090198104263406

Janega, J. B., Murray, D. M., Varnell, S. P., Blitstein, J. L., Birnbaum, A. S., & Lytle, L. A. (2004b). Assessing the most powerful analysis method for school-based intervention studies with alcohol, tobacco, and other drug outcomes. *Addictive Behaviors, 29*(3), 595–606. https://doi.org/10.1016/j.addbeh.2004.01.002

Johnson, D. B., Bruemmer, B., Lund, A. E., Evens, C. C., & Mar, C. M. (2009). Impact of school district sugar-sweetened beverage policies on student beverage exposure and consumption in middle schools. *Journal of Adolescent Health, 45*(Suppl. 3), S30–S37. https://doi.org/10.1016/j.jadohealth.2009.03.008

Kelder, S., Hoelscher, D., & Perry, C. (2015). How individuals, environments, and health behaviors interact: Social cognitive theory. In K. Glanz, B. Rimer, & K. Viswanath (Eds.), *Health behavior: Theory, research and practice* (5th ed., pp. 159–181). Jossey-Bass.

Kenny, D. A., Kashy, D. A., & Cook, W. L. (2020). *Dyadic data analysis.* Guilford Press.

Kerlinger, F. N. (1986). *Foundations of behavioral research* (3rd ed.). Holt, Rinehart and Winston.

Kilbourne, A. M., Neumann, M. S., Pincus, H. A., Bauer, M. S., & Stall, R. (2007). Implementing evidence-based interventions in health care: Application of the replicating effective programs framework. *Implementation Science, 2,* 42. https://doi.org/10.1186/1748-5908-2-42

Kingdon, J. (2011). *Agendas, alternatives, and public policies.* Pearson.

Kirk, M. A., Kelley, C., Yankey, N., Birken, S. A., Abadie, B., & Damschroder, L. (2016). A systematic review of the use of the Consolidated Framework for Implementation Research. *Implementation Science, 11*(1), 72. https://doi.org/10.1186/s13012-016-0437-z

Koller, I., Levenson, M. R., & Glück, J. (2017). What do you think you are measuring? A mixed-methods procedure for assessing the content validity of test items and theory-based scaling. *Frontiers in Psychology, 8,* 126. https://doi.org/10.3389/fpsyg.2017.00126

Krueger, R. A., & Casey, M. A. (2015). *Focus groups: A practical guide for applied research* (5th ed.). Sage Publications.

Kubik, M. Y., Lytle, L. A., & Story, M. (2001). A practical, theory-based approach to establishing school nutrition advisory councils. *Journal of the American Dietetic Association, 101*(2), 223–228. https://doi.org/10.1016/S0002-8223(01)00058-X

Lally, P., Bartle, N., & Wardle, J. (2011). Social norms and diet in adolescents. *Appetite, 57*(3), 623–627. https://doi.org/10.1016/j.appet.2011.07.015

Laska, M. N., Caspi, C. E., Lenk, K., Moe, S. G., Pelletier, J. E., Harnack, L. J., & Erickson, D. J. (2019). Evaluation of the first U.S. staple foods ordinance: Impact on nutritional quality of food store offerings, customer purchases and home food environments. *The International Journal of Behavioral Nutrition and Physical Activity, 16*(1), 83. https://doi.org/10.1186/s12966-019-0818-1

Laska, M. N., Sevcik, S. M., Moe, S. G., Petrich, C. A., Nanney, M. S., Linde, J. A., & Lytle, L. A. (2016). A 2-year young adult obesity prevention trial in the US: Process evaluation results. *Health Promotion International, 31*(4), 793–800. https://doi.org/10.1093/heapro/dav066

Lau, A. S. (2006). Making the case for selective and directed cultural adaptations of evidence-based treatments: Examples from parent training. *Clinical Psychology: Science and Practice, 13*(4), 295–310. https://doi.org/10.1111/j.1468-2850.2006.00042.x

Laverack, G. (2007). *Health promotion and practice: Building empowered communities.* McGraw Hill.

Leatherman, S., Metcalfe, M., Geissler, K., & Dunford, C. (2012). Integrating microfinance and health strategies: Examining the evidence to inform policy and practice. *Health Policy and Planning, 27*(2), 85–101. https://doi.org/10.1093/heapol/czr014

Lennertz, B., Lutzenhiser, A., & Failor, T. (2008, Summer). An introduction to charrettes. *Planning Commissioners Journal, 71,* 1–3. https://j6p3d5c7.stackpathcdn.com/wp-content/uploads/2012/07/262.pdf

Lightfoot, A. F., Thatcher, K., Simán, F. M., Eng, E., Merino, Y., Thomas, T., Coyne-Beasley, T., & Chapman, M. V. (2019). "What I wish my doctor knew about my life": Using photovoice with immigrant Latino adolescents to explore barriers to healthcare. *Qualitative Social Work: Research and Practice, 18*(1), 60–80. https://doi.org/10.1177/1473325017704034

Lorencatto, F., West, R., Stavri, Z., & Michie, S. (2013). How well is intervention content described in published reports of smoking cessation interventions? *Nicotine & Tobacco Research, 15*(7), 1273–1282. https://doi.org/10.1093/ntr/nts266

Luepker, R. V., Perry, C. L., McKinlay, S. M., Nader, P. R., Parcel, G. S., Stone, E. J., Webber, L. S., Elder, J. P., Feldman, H. A., Johnson, C. C., Kelder, S. H., Wu, M., Nader, P., Elder, J., McKenzie, T., Bachman, K., Broyles, S., Busch, E., Danna, S., . . . Verter, J. (1996). Outcomes of a field trial to improve children's dietary patterns and physical activity: The Child and Adolescent Trial for Cardiovascular Health (CATCH). *Journal of the American Medical Association, 275*(10), 768–776. https://doi.org/10.1001/jama.1996.03530340032026

Lytle, L. A. (2009). Measuring the food environment: State of the science. *American Journal of Preventive Medicine, 36*(Suppl. 4), S134–S144. https://doi.org/10.1016/j.amepre.2009.01.018

Lytle, L. A., Kelder, S. H., Perry, C. L., & Klepp, K. I. (1995). Covariance of adolescent health behaviors: The Class of 1989 Study. *Health Education Research, 10*(2), 133–146. https://doi.org/10.1093/her/10.2.133

Lytle, L. A., Kubik, M. Y., Perry, C., Story, M., Birnbaum, A. S., & Murray, D. M. (2006). Influencing healthful food choices in school and home environments: Results from the TEENS study. *Preventive Medicine, 43*(1), 8–13. https://doi.org/10.1016/j.ypmed.2006.03.020

Lytle, L. A., Laska, M. N., Linde, J. A., Moe, S. G., Nanney, M. S., Hannan, P. J., & Erickson, D. J. (2017). Weight-gain reduction among 2-year college students: The CHOICES RCT. *American Journal of Preventive Medicine, 52*(2), 183–191. https://doi.org/10.1016/j.amepre.2016.10.012

Lytle, L. A., Moe, S. G., Nanney, M. S., Laska, M. N., Linde, J. A., Petrich, C. A., & Sevcik, S. M. (2014). Designing a weight gain prevention trial for young adults: The CHOICES Study. *American Journal of Health Education, 45*(2), 67–75. https://doi.org/10.1080/19325037.2013.875962

Lytle, L. A., Murray, D. M., Perry, C. L., Story, M., Birnbaum, A. S., Kubik, M. Y., & Varnell, S. (2004). School-based approaches to affect adolescents' diets: Results from the TEENS study. *Health Education & Behavior, 31*(2), 270–287. https://doi.org/10.1177/1090198103260635

Lytle, L. A., Nicastro, H. L., Roberts, S. B., Evans, M., Jakicic, J. M., Laposky, A. D., & Loria, C. M. (2018). Accumulating Data to Optimally Predict Obesity Treatment (ADOPT) Core Measures: Behavioral domain. *Obesity, 26*(Suppl. 2), S16–S24. https://doi.org/10.1002/oby.22157

Lytle, L. A., & Perry, C. L. (2001). Applying research and theory in program planning: An example from a nutrition education intervention. *Health Promotion Practice, 2*(1), 68–80. https://doi.org/10.1177/152483990100200111

Lytle, L. A., & Sokol, R. L. (2017). Measures of the food environment: A systematic review of the field, 2007–2015. *Health & Place, 44*, 18–34. https://doi.org/10.1016/j.healthplace.2016.12.007

Lytle, L. A., Svetkey, L. P., Patrick, K., Belle, S. H., Fernandez, I. D., Jakicic, J. M., Johnson, K. C., Olson, C. M., Tate, D. F., Wing, R., & Loria, C. M. (2014). The EARLY trials: A consortium of studies targeting weight control in young adults. *Translational Behavioral Medicine, 4*(3), 304–313. https://doi.org/10.1007/s13142-014-0252-5

Lytle, L. A., Ward, J., Nader, P. R., Pedersen, S., & Williston, B. J. (2003). Maintenance of a health promotion program in elementary schools: Results from the CATCH-ON study key informant interviews. *Health Education & Behavior, 30*(4), 503–518. https://doi.org/10.1177/1090198103253655

MacLean, P. S., Rothman, A. J., Nicastro, H. L., Czajkowski, S. M., Agurs-Collins, T., Rice, E. L., Courcoulas, A. P., Ryan, D. H., Bessesen, D. H., & Loria, C. M. (2018). The Accumulating Data to Optimally Predict Obesity Treatment (ADOPT) Core Measures Project: Rationale and approach. *Obesity, 26*(Suppl. 2), S6–S15. https://doi.org/10.1002/oby.22154

Marlatt, G. A., & Donovan, D. M. (Eds.). (2005). *Relapse prevention: Maintenance strategies in the treatment of addictive behaviors* (2nd ed.). Guilford Press.

Marlatt, G. A., & Gordon, J. R. (Eds.). (1985). *Relapse prevention: Maintenance strategies in the treatment of addictive behaviors*. Guilford Press.

Marmot, M. (2015). The health gap: The challenge of an unequal world. *The Lancet, 386*(10011), 2442–2444. https://doi.org/10.1016/S0140-6736(15)00150-6

Mayne, S. L., Auchincloss, A. H., & Michael, Y. L. (2015). Impact of policy and built environment changes on obesity-related outcomes: A systematic review of naturally occurring experiments. *Obesity Reviews, 16*(5), 362–375. https://doi.org/10.1111/obr.12269

McDonald, R., Jouriles, E. N., Ramisetty-Mikler, S., Caetano, R., & Green, C. E. (2006). Estimating the number of American children living in partner-violent families. *Journal of Family Psychology, 20*(1), 137–142. https://doi.org/10.1037/0893-3200.20.1.137

McKenzie, T. L., Nader, P. R., Strikmiller, P. K., Yang, M., Stone, E. J., Perry, C. L., Taylor, W. C., Epping, J. N., Feldman, H. A., Luepker, R. V., & Kelder, S. H. (1996). School physical education: Effect of the Child and Adolescent Trial for Cardiovascular Health. *Preventive Medicine, 25*(4), 423–431. https://doi.org/10.1006/pmed.1996.0074

McKinlay, J. B., & Marceau, L. D. (1999). A tale of 3 tails. *American Journal of Public Health, 89*(3), 295–298. https://doi.org/10.2105/AJPH.89.3.295

Michie, S., Richardson, M., Johnston, M., Abraham, C., Francis, J., Hardeman, W., Eccles, M. P., Cane, J., & Wood, C. E. (2013). The behavior change technique taxonomy (v1) of 93 hierarchically clustered techniques: Building an international consensus for the reporting of behavior change interventions. *Annals of Behavioral Medicine, 46*(1), 81–95. https://doi.org/10.1007/s12160-013-9486-6

Miles, M. B., Huberman, A. M., & Saldana, J. (2014). *Qualitative data analysis: A methods sourcebook* (3rd ed.). Sage Publications.

Miller, S., Ainsworth, B., Yardley, L., Milton, A., Weal, M., Smith, P., & Morrison, L. (2019). A framework for analyzing and measuring usage and engagement date (AMUsED) in digital interventions: Viewpoint. *Journal of Medical Internet Research, 21*(2), e10966. https://doi.org/10.2196/10966

Miller-Day, M., & Hecht, M. L. (2013). Narrative means to preventative ends: A narrative engagement framework for designing prevention interventions. *Health Communication, 28*(7), 657–670. https://doi.org/10.1080/10410236.2012.762861

Minkler, M., Wallerstein, N., & Wilson, N. (2008). Improving health through community organizing and community building. In K. Glanz, B. K. Rimer, & F. M. Lewis (Eds.), *Health behavior and health education: Theory, research, and practice* (4th ed., pp. 287–312). Jossey-Bass.

Minnesota Department of Health. (n.d.). *Minnesota student survey.* https://education.mn.gov/MDE/dse/health/mss/

Moerbeek, M., & Teerenstra, S. (2016). *Power analysis of trials with multilevel data.* CRC Press.

Moher, D., Schulz, K. F., & Altman, D. G. (2001). The CONSORT statement: Revised recommendations for improving the quality of reports of parallel group randomized trials. *BMC Medical Research Methodology, 1,* Article 2. https://doi.org/10.1186/1471-2288-1-2

Montano, D. E., & Kasprzyk, D. (2015). Theory of reasoned action, theory of planned behavior and the integrated behavioral model. In K. Glanz, B. Rimer, & K. Viswanath (Eds.), *Health behavior: Theory, research, and practice* (5th ed., pp. 95–124). Jossey-Bass.

Montgomery, P., Grant, S., Mayo-Wilson, E., Macdonald, G., Michie, S., Hopewell, S., Moher, D., & the CONSORT-SPI Group. (2018). Reporting randomised trials of social and psychological interventions: The CONSORT-SPI 2018 Extension. *Trials, 19*(1), 407. https://doi.org/10.1186/s13063-018-2733-1

Moullin, J. C., Dickson, K. S., Stadnick, N. A., Albers, B., Nilsen, P., Broder-Fingert, S., Mukasa, B., & Aarons, G. A. (2020). Ten recommendations for using implementation frameworks in research and practice. *Implementation Science Communications, 1*(1), 42. https://doi.org/10.1186/s43058-020-00023-7

Moullin, J. C., Dickson, K. S., Stadnick, N. A., Rabin, B., & Aarons, G. A. (2019). Systematic review of the Exploration, Preparation, Implementation, Sustainment (EPIS) framework. *Implementation Science, 14*(1), 1. https://doi.org/10.1186/s13012-018-0842-6

Murray, D. M. (1998). *Design and analysis of group-randomized trials.* Oxford University Press.

Murray, D. M., Blitstein, J. L., Hannan, P. J., Baker, W. L., & Lytle, L. A. (2007). Sizing a trial to alter the trajectory of health behaviours: Methods, parameter estimates, and their application. *Statistics in Medicine, 26*(11), 2297–2316. https://doi.org/10.1002/sim.2714

Murray, D. M., Pennell, M., Rhoda, D., Hade, E. M., & Paskett, E. D. (2010). Designing studies that would address the multilayered nature of health care. *JNCI Monographs, 2010*(40), 90–96. https://doi.org/10.1093/jncimonographs/lgq014

Murray, D. M., Phillips, G. A., Bimbaum, A. S., & Lytle, L. A. (2001). Intraclass correlation for measures from a middle school nutrition intervention study: Estimates, correlates, and applications. *Health Education & Behavior, 28*(6), 666–679. https://doi.org/10.1177/109019810102800602

Myers, A. E., Knocke, K., & Leeman, J. (2019). Tapping into multiple data "springs" to strengthen policy streams: A guide to the types of data needed to formulate local retail tobacco control policy. *Preventing Chronic Disease, 16,* 180282. https://doi.org/10.5888/pcd16.180282

Nader, P. R., Stone, E. J., Lytle, L. A., Perry, C. L., Osganian, S. K., Kelder, S., Webber, L. S., Elder, J. P., Montgomery, D., Feldman, H. A., Wu, M., Johnson, C., Parcel, G. S., & Luepker, R. V. (1999). Three-year maintenance of improved diet and physical activity: The CATCH cohort. Child and Adolescent Trial for Cardiovascular Health. *Archives of Pediatrics & Adolescent Medicine, 153*(7), 695–704. https://doi.org/10.1001/archpedi.153.7.695

National Association of County Health Officials. (n.d.). *Model practices*. https://www.naccho.org/membership/awards/model-practices

National Cancer Institute. (n.d.). *Implementation science at a glance: A guide for cancer control practitioners*. U.S. Department of Health and Human Services (NIH Publication No. 19-CA-8055). https://cancercontrol.cancer.gov/sites/default/files/2020-07/NCI-ISaaG-Workbook.pdf

National Center for HIV/AIDS, Viral Hepatitis, STD, and TB Prevention. (n.d.). *Identifying and determining involvement of stakeholders*. Centers for Disease Control and Prevention. https://www.cdc.gov/std/Program/pupestd/Identifying%20and%20Determining%20Stakeholders.pdf

National Institutes of Health. (n.d.). *NIH planning grant program (R34)*. U.S. Department of Health & Human Services. https://grants.nih.gov/grants/funding/r34.htm

Nestle, M. (2013). *Food Politics*. University of California Press. https://doi.org/10.1525/9780520955066

Nezami, B. T., Lytle, L. A., Ward, D. S., Ennett, S. T., & Tate, D. F. (2020). Effect of the Smart Moms intervention on targeted mediators of change in child sugar-sweetened beverage intake. *Public Health*, *182*, 193–198. https://doi.org/10.1016/j.puhe.2020.03.015

Nezami, B. T., Ward, D. S., Lytle, L. A., Ennett, S. T., & Tate, D. F. (2018). A mHealth randomized controlled trial to reduce sugar-sweetened beverage intake in preschool-aged children. *Pediatric Obesity*, *13*(11), 668–676. https://doi.org/10.1111/ijpo.12258

Noar, S. M., Benac, C. N., & Harris, M. S. (2007). Does tailoring matter? Meta-analytic review of tailored print health behavior change interventions. *Psychological Bulletin*, *133*(4), 673–693. https://doi.org/10.1037/0033-2909.133.4.673

Nunnally, J. C. (1978). *Psychometric theory* (2nd ed.). McGraw-Hill.

O'Donnell, L., Stueve, A., Myint-U, A., Duran, R., Agronick, G., & Wilson-Simmons, R. (2006). Middle school aggression and subsequent intimate partner physical violence. *Journal of Youth and Adolescence*, *35*(5), 693–703. https://doi.org/10.1007/s10964-006-9086-x

Office of Disease Prevention and Health Promotion, U.S. Department of Health and Human Services. (n.d.). *Healthy People 2020: Midcourse review*. https://www.healthypeople.gov/2020/data-search/midcourse-review/lhi

Office of Disease Prevention and Health Promotion, U.S. Department of Health and Human Services. (2021). *Healthy People 2020: Evidence-based resources*. https://www.healthypeople.gov/2020/tools-resources/Evidence-Based-Resources

O'Mara-Eves, A., Brunton, G., McDaid, D., Oliver, S., Kavanagh, J., Jamal, F., Matosevic, T., Harden, A., Thomas, J., & the O-Mara-Eves. (2013). Community engagement to reduce inequalities in health: A systematic review, meta-analysis and economic analysis. *Public Health Research* (No. 1.4). NIHR Journals Library. https://doi.org/10.3310/phr01040

Osganian, S. K., Ebzery, M. K., Montgomery, D. H., Nicklas, T. A., Evans, M. A., Mitchell, P. D., Lytle, L. A., Snyder, M. P., Stone, E. J., Zive, M. M., Bachman, K. J., Rice, R., & Parcel, G. S. (1996). Changes in the nutrient content of school lunches: Results from the CATCH Eat Smart food service intervention. *Preventive Medicine*, *25*(4), 400–412. https://doi.org/10.1006/pmed.1996.0072

Parcel, G. S., Perry, C. L., Kelder, S. H., Elder, J. P., Mitchell, P. D., Lytle, L. A., Johnson, C. C., & Stone, E. J. (2003). School climate and the institutionalization of the CATCH program. *Health Education & Behavior*, *30*(4), 489–502. https://doi.org/10.1177/1090198103253650

Pearson, T. A., Wall, S., Lewis, C., Jenkins, P. L., Nafziger, A., & Weinehall, L. (2001). Dissecting the "black box" of community intervention: Lessons from community-wide cardiovascular disease prevention programs in the US and Sweden. *Scandinavian Journal of Public Health. Supplement, 56,* 69–78.

Perry, C. L. (1999). *Creating health behavior change: How to develop community-wide programs for youth.* Sage Publications.

Perry, C. L., Stone, E. J., Parcel, G. S., Ellison, R. C., Nader, P. R., Webber, L. S., & Luepker, R. V. (1990). School-based cardiovascular health promotion: The child and adolescent trial for cardiovascular health (CATCH). *The Journal of School Health, 60*(8), 406–413. https://doi.org/10.1111/j.1746-1561.1990.tb05960.x

Pew Charitable Trusts. (2021, July 20). *Results First clearinghouse database.* https://www.pewtrusts.org/en/research-and-analysis/data-visualizations/2015/results-first-clearinghouse-database

Potischman, N., & Freudenheim, J. L. (2003). Biomarkers of nutritional exposure and nutritional status: An overview. *The Journal of Nutrition, 133*(3), 873S–874S. https://doi.org/10.1093/jn/133.3.873S

Pratt, L. A., & Brody, D. J. (2014). *Depression in the U.S. household population, 2009–2012* (NCHS Data Brief, no. 172). National Center for Health Statistics.

Prochaska, J. O., Redding, C. A., & Evers, K. E. (2015). The transtheoretical model and stages of change. In K. Glanz, B. Rimer, & K. Viswanath (Eds.), *Health Behavior: Theory, Research and Practice* (5th ed., pp. 125–148). Jossey-Bass.

Proctor, E., Silmere, H., Raghavan, R., Hovmand, P., Aarons, G., Bunger, A., Griffey, R., & Hensley, M. (2011). Outcomes for implementation research: Conceptual distinctions, measurement challenges, and research agenda. *Administration and Policy in Mental Health, 38*(2), 65–76. https://doi.org/10.1007/s10488-010-0319-7

Public Policy Associates, Incorporated. (2015). *Considerations for conducting evaluation using a culturally responsive and racial equity lens.* https://publicpolicy.com/wp-content/uploads/2017/04/PPA-Culturally-Responsive-Lens.pdf

RAND Corporation. (n.d.). *RAND online measure repository.* https://www.rand.org/nsrd/ndri/centers/frp/innovative-practices/measure.html

Rogers, E. M. (2003). *Diffusion of innovations* (5th ed.). The Free Press.

Rosenbaum, M., Agurs-Collins, T., Bray, M. S., Hall, K. D., Hopkins, M., Laughlin, M., MacLean, P. S., Maruvada, P., Savage, C. R., Small, D. M., & Stoeckel, L. (2018). Accumulating Data to Optimally Predict Obesity Treatment (ADOPT): Recommendations from the biological domain. *Obesity, 26*(Suppl. 2), S25–S34. https://doi.org/10.1002/oby.22156

Rotheram-Borus, M. J., Rebchook, G. M., Kelly, J. A., Adams, J., & Neumann, M. S. (2000). Bridging research and practice: Community-researcher partnerships for replicating effective interventions. *AIDS Education and Prevention, 12*(Suppl. 5), 49–61.

Saelens, B. E., Arteaga, S. S., Berrigan, D., Ballard, R. M., Gorin, A. A., Powell-Wiley, T. M., Pratt, C., Reedy, J., & Zenk, S. N. (2018). Accumulating Data to Optimally Predict Obesity Treatment (ADOPT) Core Measures: Environmental domain. *Obesity, 26*(Suppl. 2), S35–S44. https://doi.org/10.1002/oby.22159

Sallis, J. F., Kerr, J., Carlson, J. A., Norman, G. J., Saelens, B. E., Durant, N., & Ainsworth, B. E. (2010). Evaluating a brief self-report measure of neighborhood environments for physical activity research and surveillance: Physical Activity Neighborhood Environment Scale (PANES). *Journal of Physical Activity & Health,* 7(4), 533–540. https://doi.org/10.1123/jpah.7.4.533

Samuel, C. A., Lightfoot, A. F., Schaal, J., Yongue, C., Black, K., Ellis, K., Robertson, L., Smith, B., Jones, N., Foley, K., Kollie, J., Mayhand, A., Morse, C., Guerrab, F., & Eng, E. (2018). Establishing new community-based participatory research partnerships using the community-based participator research charrette model: Lessons from the Caner Health Accountability for Managing Pain and Symptoms study. *Progress in Community Health Partnerships, 12*(1), 89–99. https://doi.org/10.1353/cpr.2018.0010

Saris, W. E., & Gallhofer, I. N. (2014). *Design, evaluation, and analysis of questionnaires for survey research* (2nd ed.). John Wiley and Sons. https://doi.org/10.1002/9781118634646

Schoeller, D. A. (1995). Limitations in the assessment of dietary energy intake by self-report. *Metabolism: Clinical and Experimental, 44*(2, Suppl. 2), 18–22. https://doi.org/10.1016/0026-0495(95)90204-X

Schoeny, M. E., Fogg, L., Buchholz, S. W., Miller, A., & Wilbur, J. (2017). Barriers to physical activity as moderators of intervention effects. *Preventive Medicine Reports, 5*, 57–64. https://doi.org/10.1016/j.pmedr.2016.11.008

Schulz, K. F., Altman, D. G., Moher, D., & the CONSORT Group. (2010). CONSORT 2010 statement: Updated guidelines for reporting parallel group randomised trials. *British Medical Journal, 340*(2), c332. https://doi.org/10.1136/bmj.c332

Shadish, W. R., Cook, T. D., & Campbell, D. T. (2002). *Experimental and quasi-experimental designs for generalized causal inference*. Houghton, Mifflin, and Company.

Skinner, B. F. (1938). *The behavior of organisms*. Appleton-Century-Crofts.

Skinner, C. S., Tiro, J., & Champion, V. L. (2015). The health belief model. In K. Glanz, B. Rimer, & K. Viswanath (Eds.), *Health behavior: Theory, research and practice* (5th ed., pp. 75–94). Jossey-Bass.

Smith, S., Winkler, S., Towne, S., & Lutz, B. (2020). Utilizing CBPR charrette in community–academic research partnerships—What stakeholders should know. *Journal of Participatory Research Methods, 1*(1). Advance online publication. https://doi.org/10.35844/001c.13179

Spencer, L., Pagell, F., Hallion, M. E., & Adams, T. B. (2002). Applying the trans-theoretical model to tobacco cessation and prevention: A review of literature. *American Journal of Health Promotion, 17*(1), 7–71. https://doi.org/10.4278/0890-1171-17.1.7

Steckler, A., & Linnan, L. (Eds.). (2002). *Process evaluation for public health inter-ventions and research*. Jossey-Bass.

Stevens, J., Murray, D. M., Catellier, D. J., Hannan, P. J., Lytle, L. A., Elder, J. P., Young, D. R., Simons-Morton, D. G., & Webber, L. S. (2005). Design of the Trial of Activity in Adolescent Girls (TAAG). *Contemporary Clinical Trials, 26*(2), 223–233. https://doi.org/10.1016/j.cct.2004.12.011

Stevens, J., Pratt, C., Boyington, J., Nelson, C., Truesdale, K. P., Ward, D. S., Lytle, L., Sherwood, N. E., Robinson, T. N., Moore, S., Barkin, S., Cheung, Y. K., & Murray, D. M. (2017). Multilevel interventions targeting obesity: Research recommendations for vulnerable populations. *American Journal of Preventive Medicine, 52*(1), 115–124. https://doi.org/10.1016/j.amepre.2016.09.011

Story, M., Kaphingst, K. M., Robinson-O'Brien, R., & Glanz, K. (2008). Creating healthy food and eating environments: Policy and environmental approaches. *Annual Review of Public Health, 29*(1), 253–272. https://doi.org/10.1146/annurev.publhealth.29.020907.090926

Story, M., Lytle, L. A., Birnbaum, A. S., & Perry, C. L. (2002). Peer-led, school-based nutrition education for young adolescents: Feasibility and process evaluation of the TEENS study. *The Journal of School Health, 72*(3), 121–127. https://doi.org/10.1111/j.1746-1561.2002.tb06529.x

Streiner, D. L., & Norman, G. R. (2003). *Health measurement scales: A practical guide to their development and use* (3rd ed.). Oxford University Press.

Strimbu, K., & Tavel, J. A. (2010). What are biomarkers? *Current Opinion in HIV and AIDS, 5*(6), 463–466. https://doi.org/10.1097/COH.0b013e32833ed177

Substance Abuse and Mental Health Services Administration. (n.d.). *Evidence-based practices resource center.* U.S. Department of Health & Human Services. https://www.samhsa.gov/resource-search/ebp

Sutin, A. R., Boutelle, K., Czajkowski, S. M., Epel, E. S., Green, P. A., Hunter, C. M., Rice, E. L., Williams, D. M., Young-Hyman, D., & Rothman, A. J. (2018). Accumulating Data to Optimally Predict Obesity Treatment (ADOPT) Core Measures: Psychosocial domain. *Obesity, 26*(Suppl. 2), S45–S54. https://doi.org/10.1002/oby.22160

Swank, J. M., & Mullen, P. R. (2017). Evaluating evidence for conceptually related constructs using bivariate correlations. *Measurement & Evaluation in Counseling & Development, 50*(4), 270–274. https://doi.org/10.1080/07481756.2017.1339562

Taplin, S. H., Anhang Price, R., Edwards, H. M., Foster, M. K., Breslau, E. S., Chollette, V., Prabhu Das, I., Clauser, S. B., Fennell, M. L., & Zapka, J. (2012). Introduction: Understanding and influencing multilevel factors across the cancer care continuum. *JNCI Monographs, 2012*(44), 2–10. https://doi.org/10.1093/jncimonographs/lgs008

Thaler, R. H., & Sunstein, C. R. (2008). *Nudge: Improving decisions about health, wealth, and happiness.* Yale University Press.

Tolley, E. E., Ulin, P. R., Mack, N., Robinson, E. T., & Succop, S. M. (2016). *Qualitative methods in public health: A field guide for applied research* (2nd ed.). Jossey-Bass.

Truong, W., & Aronne, L. J. (2018). ADOPT: Obesity treatment reaches level of maturity with its own collaborative initiative and resource. *Obesity, 26*(Suppl. 2), S5. https://doi.org/10.1002/oby.22181

UNICEF. (2017). *Report on communication for development (C4D). Global progress and country level highlights across programme areas.* https://www.unicef.org/media/47781/file/UNICEF_2017_Report_on_Communication_for_Development_C4D.pdf

U.S. Department of Agriculture. (2020). *Dietary guidelines for Americans, 2020–2025* (9th ed.). U.S. Department of Health and Human Services. https://www.dietaryguidelines.gov/sites/default/files/2020-12/Dietary_Guidelines_for_Americans_2020-2025.pdf

U.S. Department of Health and Human Services. (2018). *Physical activity guidelines for Americans* (2nd ed.). U.S. Department of Health and Human Services. https://health.gov/sites/default/files/2019-09/Physical_Activity_Guidelines_2nd_edition.pdf

U.S. Department of Health and Human Services' Physical Activity Guidelines Advisory Committee. (2018). *2018 Physical Activity Guidelines Advisory Committee scientific report.* U.S. Department of Health and Human Services. https://health.gov/our-work/physical-activity/current-guidelines/scientific-report

U.S. National Cancer Institute. (n.d.). *Evidence-based cancer control programs.* https://ebccp.cancercontrol.cancer.gov/index.do

U.S. Preventive Service Task Force. (n.d.). *New recommendation: Screening for pre-diabetes and Type 2 diabetes.* https://uspreventiveservicestaskforce.org/uspstf/

Valente, T. W. (2015). Social networks and health behavior. In K. Glanz, B. Rimer, & K. Viswanath (Eds.), *Health behavior: Theory, research and practice* (5th ed., pp. 205–222). Jossey-Bass.

Wadden, T. A., West, D. S., Delahanty, L., Jakicic, J., Rejeski, J., Williamson, D., Berkowitz, R. I., Kelley, D. E., Tomchee, C., Hill, J. O., Kumanyika, S., & the Look AHEAD Research Group. (2006). The Look AHEAD study: A description of the lifestyle intervention and the evidence supporting it. *Obesity, 14*(5), 737–752. https://doi.org/10.1038/oby.2006.84

Wallerstein, N. (1994). Empowerment education applied to youth. In A. C. Matiella (Ed.), *Multicultural challenge in health education* (pp. 153–176). ETR Associates.

Wallerstein, N., Minkler, M., Carter-Edwards, L., Avila, M., & Sanchez, V. (2015). Improving health through community engagement, community organization and community building. In K. Glanz, B. Rimer, & K. Viswanath (Eds.), *Health behavior: Theory, research and practice* (5th ed., pp. 227–300). Jossey-Bass.

Watson, J. B. (1925). *Behaviorism.* Norton.

Webber, L. S., Catellier, D. J., Lytle, L. A., Murray, D. M., Pratt, C. A., Young, D. R., Elder, J. P., Lohman, T. G., Stevens, J., Jobe, J. B., Pate, R. R., & the TAAG Collaborative Research Group. (2008). Promoting physical activity in middle school girls: Trial of Activity for Adolescent Girls. *American Journal of Preventive Medicine, 34*(3), 173–184. https://doi.org/10.1016/j.amepre.2007.11.018

Weinstein, N. D. (2007). Misleading tests of health behavior theories. *Annals of Behavioral Medicine, 33*(1), 1–10. https://doi.org/10.1207/s15324796abm3301_1

Weiss, E. C., Galuska, D. A., Kettel Khan, L., Gillespie, C., & Serdula, M. K. (2007). Weight regain in U.S. adults who experienced substantial weight loss, 1999–2002. *American Journal of Preventive Medicine, 33*(1), 34–40. https://doi.org/10.1016/j.amepre.2007.02.040

Whitehead, A. L., Sully, B. G. O., & Campbell, M. J. (2014). Pilot and feasibility studies: Is there a difference from each other and from a randomised controlled trial? *Contemporary Clinical Trials, 38*(1), 130–133. https://doi.org/10.1016/j.cct.2014.04.001

Wilbur, J., Miller, A. M., Fogg, L., McDevitt, J., Castro, C. M., Schoeny, M. E., Buchholz, S. W., Braun, L. T., Ingram, D. M., Volgman, A. S., & Dancy, B. L. (2016). Randomized clinical trial of the women's lifestyle physical activity program for African-American women: 24 and 48 week outcomes. *American Journal of Health Promotion, 30*(5), 335–345. Advance online publication. https://doi.org/10.1177/0890117116646342

Wiltsey Stirman, S., Baumann, A. A., & Miller, C. J. (2019). The FRAME: An expanded framework for reporting adaptations and modifications to evidence-based interventions. *Implementation Science; IS, 14*(1), 58. https://doi.org/10.1186/s13012-019-0898-y

World Health Organization. (n.d.). *The VPA approach.* https://www.who.int/groups/violence-prevention-alliance/approach

Young, D. R., Johnson, C. C., Steckler, A., Gittelsohn, J., Saunders, R. P., Saksvig, B. I., Ribisl, K. M., Lytle, L. A., & McKenzie, T. L. (2006). Data to action: Using formative research to develop intervention programs to increase physical activity in adolescent girls. *Health Education & Behavior, 33*(1), 97–111. https://doi.org/10.1177/1090198105282444

Young, D. R., Steckler, A., Cohen, S., Pratt, C., Felton, G., Moe, S. G., Pickrel, J., Johnson, C. C., Grieser, M., Lytle, L. A., Lee, J. S., & Raburn, B. (2008). Process evaluation results from a school- and community-linked intervention: The Trial of Activity for Adolescent Girls (TAAG). *Health Education Research, 23*(6), 976–986. https://doi.org/10.1093/her/cyn029

Yu, D. L., & Seligman, M. E. P. (2002). Preventing depressive symptoms in Chinese children. *Prevention & Treatment, 5*(1), 9. https://doi.org/10.1037/1522-3736.5.1.59a

Zyphur, M. J., Zhang, Z., Preacher, K. F., & Bird, L. (2019). Moderated mediation in multilevel structural equation models. In S. E. Humphrey & J. M. LeBreton (Eds.), *The handbook of multilevel theory, measurement, and analysis* (pp. 473–494). American Psychological Association. https://doi.org/10.1037/0000115-021

INDEX

ABOUT THE AUTHOR

Leslie Ann Lytle, PhD, is an adjunct professor of health behavior and an adjunct professor of nutrition at the Gillings School of Global Public Health, University of North Carolina (UNC) at Chapel Hill. She is also an adjunct professor in the Division of Epidemiology and Community Health at the University of Minnesota, Minneapolis. Her research over the past 30 years has centered on designing, conducting, and evaluating multilevel interventions to promote community health with a focus on health promotion of youth and young adults, particularly preventing obesity and promoting healthful diet and physical activity through school, family, and environmental approaches. Dr. Lytle's research portfolio includes intervention trials as well as etiologic studies examining multilevel determinants of health behaviors. She has been the principal investigator on several large National Institutes of Health (NIH) studies, including CATCH (National Heart, Lung, and Blood Institute [NHLBI]), TEENS (National Cancer Institute [NCI]), TAAG (NHLBI), IDEA (NCI), ECHO (NHLBI), and CHOICES (NHLBI), and she has participated as a coinvestigator in many other community-based studies. She has published more than 240 articles in the peer-reviewed literature and has served on many expert panels for the NIH and the Centers for Disease Control and Prevention.

Dr. Lytle received a BS in medical dietetics from Pennsylvania State University and a master's in education from Purdue University. Her doctoral degree in health behavior and health education is from the University of Michigan. Before joining UNC, she was on the faculty of the Division of Epidemiology and Community Health in the University of Minnesota's School of Public Health for more than 20 years. Dr. Lytle has taught courses in theories of health behavior change, community nutrition interventions, and behavioral and social aspects of health.